ALSO BY JOANNE LAMB HAYES

Grandma's Wartime Kitchen

WITH BONNIE TANDY LEBLANG

Grains
Beans
365 Great Cookies and Brownies
The Weekend Kitchen
Rice
Country Entertaining

CONTRIBUTOR

McCall's No Time to Cook
The Gingerbread Book
The New Revised and Updated McCall's Cookbook

Recipes from America's Small Farms

Recipes from America's Small Farms

Fresh Ideas for the Season's Bounty

Joanne Lamb Hayes and Lori Stein
with Maura Webber

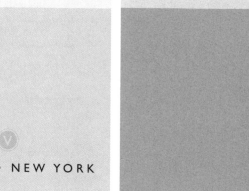

VILLARD · NEW YORK

2003 Villard Books Trade Paperback Original

The following recipes were reprinted with permission:
Green Soup (Caldo Verde), from *The Food of Portugal,* by Jean Anderson, © 1986 by Jean Anderson,
reprinted by permission of HarperCollins Publishers, Inc.
Dandelion Columbo, from *The Wild Vegetarian Cookbook,* by Steve Brill, © 2002 by Steve Brill,
reprinted by permission of Harvard Common Press.

Library of Congress Cataloging-in-Publication Data

Recipes from America's small farms : fresh ideas for the season's bounty /
Joanne Lamb Hayes and Lori Stein with Maura Webber.
p.   cm.
Includes index.
ISBN 0-8129-6775-5
1. Cookery, American. I. Hayes, Joanne Lamb. II. Stein, Lori. III. Webber, Maura.
TX715 .R31213 2003
641.5973—dc21   2002191052

Villard Books website address: www.villard.com

Printed in the United States of America

2 4 6 8 9 7 5 3 1

Book design by Carole Lowenstein

ACKNOWLEDGMENTS

We would like to thank the following people whose help made this book possible:

Angela Miller, our agent, for finding it the perfect home
Mary Bahr, our editor, whose passion for the project made it fun
Andrew Levine, for the cover photography
Claire H. Lewis, for the author photo
Deena Stein, for proofreading anytime, day or night
Michelle Stein, for computer support whenever we needed it
Bonnie Lane Webber, for so much great advice
The CSA farmers who sent their recipes at the height of the harvest season
Nancy Civetta, for bringing us together with the chefs of Chefs Collaborative
The chefs of Chefs Collaborative, for their recipes and enthusiastic support
Pat Foo and Ken Holtz, for the cover location
Jim Angelucci of Phillips Mushrooms, for the cover basket collection
Stephanie Reph of the Robin Van En Center, for CSA Resources
Benjamin Dreyer, who made sure the book was properly edited
Testers Tanya Furtado, Bonnie Webber, Kate Learson, Deb Palmer, Edith Harnik, Deena Stein, Michelle Stein, Shelly Katz Biederman, Becca Cherry
All the volunteers at our site: Stephanie Margolin, Steve Waxman, Roberto Adsuar, Manuela Pizzi, Alan Brown, Jenni and Pete Cosenza

CONTENTS

INTRODUCTION

Every Tuesday afternoon, a crowd gathers on a busy Manhattan street corner, watching for the big white truck that soon arrives. A brigade forms to unload crate after crate of gorgeous, fragrant vegetables: bright orange cherry tomatoes (luckily, we're allowed to eat just a few as we unpack, because their aroma is irresistible), delicate fingerling potatoes, tiny striped squash, teardrop-shaped cabbages, big-as-a-penny raspberries, and basil that is as potent as perfume.

As we fill our bags with the visibly fresh produce, passersby, lured by sight and scent, stop and ask, "What's going on here?" We explain that Tuesday is CSA day, that all of us are members of a Community Supported Agriculture project. In the spring, we bought shares in the harvest of Stoneledge Farm, a small certified organic farm located about two hours north of our neighborhood. Now, from June to November, we receive our bounty. Every week, our farmers harvest all the vegetables that are ready, and bring them to this central location for us to pick up. Every week's share is a surprise package, always fresh, always delicious.

By itself, this little scene wouldn't make much of a difference to the overall health of the environment or to the farming community. But it's being repeated in more than a thousand locations in the United States each week, supporting more than a thousand small farms whose very existence would be threatened without their shareholders. And the movement is growing every year. As Alice Waters, chef of Chez Panisse, has said, "Community Supported Agriculture is the most positive-spirited movement in the country today."

The CSA concept originated in Japan almost forty years ago by mothers who wanted a more personal connection to their food source; they called their farm-to-consumer co-ops *teikei,* which translates roughly to "food with a face on it." In 1985, the first American CSA was organized in South Egremont, Massachusetts, by Robyn Van En, a food activist. For the next decade, the movement grew slowly; then in the late 1990s, it took off as people became more aware of and interested in food issues, and as many of them became determined to buy food that was produced by nearby, responsible farmers.

There's no overall organization of CSAs, no governing body; each group makes its own way and its own rules. Some CSAs require members to volunteer their time; others simply deliver to each member's door. Some offer only vegetables; others include fruit, meat, dairy, honey, and other products. Some have fewer than a dozen members; others have hundreds. But the idea is the same: Farmers and communities join together to support each other so that the communities can receive the freshest, most nutritious, and tastiest produce available, and so that the farmers—knowing that their crops are sold—can concentrate on farming as safely and as well as they can without worrying about marketing.

Why do we do it? Why do so many people from every economic, ethnic, and educational level take the time and make the effort to get their food through CSA when it is so much more conveniently available and neatly packaged on supermarket shelves? And why do so many farmers complicate their already demanding profession by connecting themselves with a mass of members rather than with a few wholesalers? Part of the reason that CSA has grown so rapidly is that the food tastes so much better. Zucchini just pulled from the vine have a sweet tenderness that is utterly lacking in those that have made a five-day trip in a refrigerated van. Onions that arrive still encrusted in soil are stronger and richer tasting than the ones that have been sitting in supermarket barrels for months. CSA farmers are able to provide varieties that are too fragile to ship by conventional methods. "It's not uncommon for people to say, 'I haven't tasted a tomato like this since my grandmother grew it in her backyard,' " says Laurel Shouvlin of Bluebird Hills Farm in Springfield, Ohio.

Health is another factor. We all know that vegetables are good for us, but the nutritional value of vegetables begins to decline as soon as they are picked; so the fresher your food, the more nutritious it is. Linda Nash of Sunflower Fields Family Farm in Postville, Iowa, says that huge conventional farms "can never sell something to someone that was picked fresh that morning. That's what I can do." Besides, the varieties that are bred for easy growing and for transportability are not the ones that are best for us. "That pink, cottony tomato has had all the good stuff bred out of it, both vitamins and taste," says Terra Brockman of Henry's Farm in Congerville, Illinois.

For many, CSA is about the mutually rewarding connection between farmer and consumer. John Peterson of Angelic Organics in Caledonia, Illinois, says, "There's something about knowing the people who get the food; the cycle is expanded from seed to final use and it makes farming more vital." Those who join CSA do so because they want to bring a connection to the earth back into their lives, because they don't want their children growing up with the notion that food comes from supermarkets. Susan Zacharakis-Jutz of Local Harvest CSA, in Solon, Ohio, loves to hear parents tell their children, "That's our farmer." One CSA member from New York told us, "We like knowing when our carrots go into the ground, when our tomatoes start to ripen—we don't even mind doing without a particular vegetable when it is hit by bad weather or bugs."

CSA members learn to enjoy the rhythm of the seasons, to wait for the first tender greens and peas of spring, to savor the first fruits of summer, to preserve the heavy, flavorful squash and root vegetables of autumn. Eating with the seasons means that you don't have broccoli in August or peppers in June—but once you taste the broccoli of October or the peppers of August, the sacrifice is well rewarded!

But the pleasure of today's meal is only part of CSA's reason for being and for its success. As CSA members, we support small local farms because we know that they are critical to life and that they are endangered. Thousands of small farms go out of business every year. The huge farms that grow almost all the food in our supermarkets are certainly more efficient, but their farming practices create environmental hazards that we're not willing to accept. "It's important that we remain in touch with our land—you have to have time to walk outside and really look at your soil—and the bigger you get, the less likely that is to happen," says Susan Zacharakis-Jutz. Large corporations are concerned mostly with their bottom lines, and if we allow all the small farms to go out of business, we will have no choice but to eat the food that these corporations think we should eat—food that has been genetically modified, bred for transportability (food in the United States travels an average of thirteen hundred miles from the farm to the market shelf), and fertilized and sprayed with lethal chemicals that will stay in our soil for hundreds of years. Even the organic segment of the market is being taken over by agribusiness. If we don't want to hand over our food to corporations, we have to support the people who will grow it the way we want it grown.

Recipes from America's Small Farms was created by and for CSA members, but also for the general public, for those of you who know somewhere in the back of your mind that you need to be involved in keeping the food chain safe and local but don't know how to start. Because of our common vision, Chefs Collaborative members have generously contributed their recipes and their thoughts to this project. We hope that this book will help CSA expand, both because a part of the profits will be donated to organizations that foster the

About Chefs Collaborative

People who love and know food are among the strongest supporters of CSA; that's why responsible and enlightened chefs have embraced the CSA movement and why Chefs Collaborative has contributed dozens of recipes to this book. Chefs Collaborative is a national network of more than a thousand members of the food community who promote sustainable cuisine by celebrating the joys of local, seasonal cooking and recognizing the impact of food on our lives, our communities, and the global environment. Founded in 1993, Chefs Collaborative provides its members with tools for running economically healthy food-service establishments and making environmentally sound decisions. The national group sponsors conferences, seminars, and tastings and publishes newsletters and chefs' guides. Local chapters allow regional groups to come together and address issues of importance to their communities: Portland members teach cooking lessons to more than fifty classrooms in their community; Philadelphia members have identified sources of non–genetically modified food for their restaurants. Chefs Collaborative believes that encouraging sustainable practices will improve the quality and taste of the food we eat. That's why it is dedicated to preserving local growers who enrich communities by providing distinctive seasonal produce to both individuals and restaurants and who practice conservation methods that lessen the impact of agriculture on the environment. Chefs Collaborative recipes, which you'll find throughout this book, show the network's love of food and its desire to spread that passion to the public.

CSA movement and because it will help spread the word about CSA and the importance of responsible farming.

Every recipe in this book has been tested by food professionals; we used exactly the ingredients listed and carefully measured or weighed each one as necessary. So if you take these recipes and follow them diligently, you will get the same results as we did. But remember, though every one of these recipes will yield a delicious dish, they won't be as rewarding as the ones you create yourself from whatever is freshest. Other than in the recipes for baked goods (which need to be strictly followed so that the chemical reactions required for baking occur), we encourage you to substitute and make changes with abandon—because the best way of cooking with fresh vegetables is to let the

Organic, Sustainable, Biodiversity: What and Why?

Community Supported Agriculture is closely connected to organic and sustainable agriculture. What do these terms mean? Organic farmers don't use chemical fertilizers or pesticides. Instead, they've developed an arsenal of environmentally friendly methods to enrich their soil and avoid insect damage. Compost—decomposed plant matter and animal waste—is a favorite soil amendment; fish, kelp, and other marine products are also used. Organic farmers also often use cover crops: certain crops, like clover and alfalfa, add tons of valuable nitrogen to the soil. To reduce insect populations, these farmers grow resistant varieties, rotate crops so that pests that gravitate to specific plantings are displaced every season, attract beneficial insects (those that prey on destructive "bad" bugs) by providing plants that the "good" bugs like, and use nontoxic, plant-based insecticides. Until recently, the term "organic" had no official definition. In 1999, Congress passed the Organic Standards Act, which requires all products that are called organic to pass specific criteria and to be inspected by impartial certification agents (you'll see their stamps, such as NOFA [for Northeast Organic Farming Association] and OREGON TILTH, on organic products). There's been great debate about the usefulness and fairness of these organic standards; see page 263 for more information.

Almost all CSA farms also promote biodiversity, by planting a wide variety of crops. Commercial farms often plant huge swaths of a single variety (monocropping). Monocropping promotes pests and disease—once pests dig into a thousand acres of a crop they like, they'll stay until they're chased away with lethal chemicals. A diverse planting gives the farmer insurance against the need for that kind of control—if a bug attacks one kind of squash, the farmer still has six other kinds. Biodiversity also retains a healthy gene pool; every time a plant disappears because farmers have concentrated on more popular, easier-to-grow types, we lose not only that plant (which is often more flavorful than its more convenient cousins) but also all the desirable properties that could be bred from it.

Organic and biodiverse methods allow sustainable agriculture, the ability of a farm to grow by using its own resources. As Henry Brockman of Henry's Farm in Congerville, Illinois, says, "Commercial farms might be able to provide for the needs of this generation, but seven generations down the line, they're going to run out of the chemical products they depend upon after they deplete the soil and eliminate natural pest controls. The sustainable farm will continue to thrive because it relies on products that it produces itself, and because it enriches the world around it."

harvest inspire you. Chapter 1 of this book presents basic techniques; chapter 2 gives you basic recipes that can be adapted to whatever is growing right now in your region. And we have, of course, presented hundreds of finished dishes, tried-and-true combinations. We've tried to include something for everyone and for every occasion, for the times when you have fifteen minutes to put dinner on the table and don't intend to use more than one pot, and for the days when you're fully willing to spend ten dollars for a tiny bottle of Champagne vinegar because it will make the meal just a little more special. Some of our recipes use very little fat and contain very few calories; others, which you'll probably want to use less frequently, are pure indulgence. But if a recipe calls for spinach and you have a lovely bunch of chard, just use what you have. Add your favorite herbs and just leave out the ones you don't much like. If you prefer Parmesan cheese to feta (or if you have some Parmesan left over), then Parmesan it is. We've provided the inspiration; just add imagination and stir well!

And most important, support your local farms—by becoming a CSA member, by buying at farmers' markets and roadside stands, by encouraging the stores in which you shop to buy from nearby farms. If we don't support our farms, we're going to lose them! And there's no recipe that will make up for that.

Recipes from America's Small Farms

CHAPTER ONE

BASIC TECHNIQUES

As they are picking up their weekly shares, CSA members often ask us how to clean, store, and use the vegetables. The volunteers working at the site always share their knowledge of the vegetables in question, but tips are immediately added by other members who have come to pick up their produce. We try to make a note of some of this advice and include it in our weekly newsletters. Because members come from all over the world as well as from all over the United States, it is exciting to hear the many different ways a particular vegetable can be handled. This chapter incorporates much of the basics we have learned, while tips for handling specific vegetables will be found in the recipe chapters that follow. We love fresh vegetables because they contribute color, flavor, texture, and nutrition to our diet. All of those factors are affected by the way we handle, store, and cook our produce. These guidelines will help you decide what to do next when you arrive home with a variety of fresh organic vegetables and will provide options when you have no plans for dinner.

One of the major advantages of membership in a CSA is that you have a ready, summer-long supply of local vegetables that have been picked at their prime and shipped a very short distance, and not been warehoused before you get them. This in itself ensures better flavor and less deterioration than in produce that has been picked underripe, shipped across the country, and stored in a wholesale market before reaching your supermarket. To keep your produce in good condition once you get it home, you need to do three things: reduce its respiration, prevent dehydration, and reduce bacterial and

Cleaning and Storing Vegetables

Banning Browning

Each group of pigments in fruits and vegetables lives by its own special set of rules. Chlorophyll-related compounds, those that produce green, and the anthocyanins, those that produce reds and purples, change color in acidic and basic environments. But the most annoying of these special rules is that of flavonoids, which, with the help of enzymes, interact with oxygen and cause browning in foods such as apples, apricots, avocados, bananas, cherries, eggplant, mushrooms, peaches, pears, potatoes, and sweet potatoes. Although different varieties of the flavonoid-containing foods experience oxidation to a different degree, and plant breeders continue to develop varieties that are more resistant to browning, it is best to plan ahead and have one of the following remedies ready before you start to peel or slice and expose one of these foods to oxygen:

Eliminate Oxygen: Have a bowl of cool water ready and submerge the fruit or vegetable in it as soon as you peel, slice, or shred it. If the water starts to discolor, drain it and replace it with fresh water.

Use an Antioxidant: Shredded onion or acidic juices such as lemon juice, orange juice, and tomato juice are usually the best choices. If none of those flavors pair with what you are making, you will find powdered antioxidants made especially for this in the canning-supply section of your supermarket. Ascorbic acid and salt water will also work.

Deactivate the Enzymes: If you are going to cook the fruit or vegetable anyway or if blanching won't make it less suitable for the purpose you have in mind, a plunge into boiling water stops the action of the enzymes on the surface of the food.

mold activity. Even after harvest, vegetables continue to take in oxygen and release carbon dioxide, and this means that they continue their cycle of maturation, which eventually leads to deterioration. Chilling them slows their metabolic activity and prolongs freshness. Covering them tightly helps to reduce the available oxygen and prevent dehydration but may provide the perfect environment for mold growth and doesn't allow the carbon dioxide to escape.

Vegetables will keep longer if they aren't rinsed until you are ready to use them, but they can still be trimmed and placed in paper or plastic bags so that they will take up less room in the refrigerator. As a general rule, refrigerator storage in a "breathable" bag (muslin, brown paper, one of the special plastic bags that have tiny holes, or a regular bag with a few holes snipped into it) and periodic removal of any spots or deteriorating pieces will prolong vegetable quality. However, each recipe chapter includes specifics for the vegetables included there. Onions, tomatoes, and potatoes are notable exceptions to this storage rule and should be stored at room temperature, each for a different reason (see chapters 5, 8, and 9).

Some CSA members find it more convenient to rinse all their produce the day they get it, so that it is ready to use in a hurry for the rest of the week. If you do choose to do this, be sure to drain the vegetables well and plan to use the leafy ones within a few days. Leafy vegetables will keep longer if dried in a salad spinner or wrapped in a kitchen towel after rinsing; root vegetables and fruit vegetables such as tomatoes, squash, and peppers can be allowed to air dry before storing.

We are often asked if it is really necessary to rinse our produce, since it is all organic. Although such produce has no pesticide or chemical fertilizer residue on it, we still recommend rinsing it. Any sand or soil clinging to leaves and roots needs to be removed, and the "tiny footprints" of birds, small animals, and insects who may have visited the fields should be rinsed away. You might have noticed that we never say "wash" the vegetables. We did once and were asked, "With soap?" No, no, no; just a rinse in fresh, cool water will be fine.

Preparing Raw Vegetables

Most of the vegetables in our shares don't need to be cooked at all. The exceptions are shelled and dried beans, beets, brussels sprouts, eggplant, parsnips, potatoes, salsify, and winter squash. Even kohlrabi, turnips, and rutabagas can be eaten raw if they are shredded or thinly sliced. Slice, dice, or shred vegetables as near as possible to the time you will eat them; they begin to deteriorate, discolor due to oxidation (see Banning Browning, page 4), dry out on the surface, and lose nutrients as soon as they are cut. If you are preparing crudités for a crowd and must cut and arrange raw vegetables in advance, select those that do not oxidize. Broccoli, carrots, cauliflower, cherry tomatoes, cucumbers, kohlrabi, peppers, radishes, rutabagas, green beans, tomatoes, and turnips make great crudités. Prepare and arrange them on the serving platter, cover them with moistened cheesecloth and plastic wrap, then refrigerate them until just before serving. If you are including tomatoes, the flavor will be better if you slice them, cover them tightly, and set them aside at room temperature; add them to the platter just before serving. If you are cutting or shredding something that oxidizes, toss the pieces immediately with an acid such as lemon, orange, or tomato juice, shredded onion, vinegar, salad dressing, yogurt, sour cream, or a vitamin C tablet dissolved in water, to prevent darkening.

Raw vegetables make wonderful natural containers for dips, sauces, spreads, salad dressings, soups, stews, or salads. Depending upon the size container you need, remove the top and clean or hollow out the center of a summer or winter squash, pumpkin, pepper, tomato, or cabbage. Once it has served as a container, you can rinse and cook the hollowed-out vegetable for another use. Raw vegetables make perfect garnishes. Anything from simple sprigs of flowering herbs to intricately crafted vegetable flowers can be added to individual plates or serving trays or platters to enhance their appearance. (See Some Easy Garnishes, page 8.)

Cooking Vegetables

BOILING: Until recently, American cooks had a tendency to boil all their vegetables, and, in many cases, to overboil them until they had lost all identity. Boiling provides a steady temperature (212°F), plenty of moisture, and, unless all the water boils away, insurance against burning. A general guideline for boiling vegetables is to bring just enough water to a boil to cover the vegetables. Add the vegetables, return to a boil, and then start timing according to the individual recipe. An old-fashioned way to get this right is to boil the water in a teakettle, put the vegetables in the saucepan, and pour in just the right amount of boiling water from the kettle to cover them. Tender vegetables such as corn, green beans, and broccoli can take as little as 3 to 5 minutes. Tough vegetables such as large beets, turnips, and sweet potatoes can take 30 minutes or more. It is important to take vegetables out of the water when they are crisp-tender because they will cook a bit more from their residual heat on the way to the table. Using a lid contains the heat, causing the water to come to a boil faster and the vegetables to cook more quickly. Be sure to follow the recipe directions for heat intensity, for whether to use a cover or not, and for timing. A lid is a good idea for vegetables that need a longer cooking time, but it can overcook fragile vegetables, such as asparagus and green beans, in a hurry. The rule for vegetable boiling used to be to use little water and a lid for mild-flavored vegetables, such as carrots and peas, and lots of water and no lid for strong-flavored ones, such as onions and cabbage. But these days people have come to appreciate the vibrant flavors of vegetables such as onions and cabbage, and using extra water to get rid of their flavor is a thing of the past.

BRAISING: Braising is a technique borrowed from meat cookery. It is especially good for roots and tubers because the long, slow heating in a minimum of liquid enhances their flavor as it inches them toward tenderness. To braise vegetables, heat a fat such as butter, olive oil, or vegetable oil in a heavy skillet or Dutch oven. Add the vegetables and cook them, stirring frequently, until they begin to brown. Add a little broth, water, wine, or fruit juice; cover the skillet; and cook the vegetables slowly over low heat until they are just tender. If there is still liquid in the skillet, simmer the vegetables, uncovered, until enough liquid evaporates to form a thickened glaze. If you don't want to keep an eye on the skillet to make sure there is still enough liquid to prevent scorching, you can use an ovenproof skillet and lid and braise the vegetables in a 325°F oven.

BROILING: There is nothing more attuned to today's busy lifestyle than broiling. Even CSA farmers have times when they need to make dinner in minutes, and this is the way to do it. Broiling is the indoor equivalent of grilling, except the foods are cooked under instead of over an intense, direct heat source. You can brush slices of summer or winter squash, eggplant, asparagus, broccoli, cauliflower, onion, and much more with olive oil, salad dressing, or a marinade and broil them for 3 to 5 minutes. Turn them, brush them again, and broil them until they are just crisp-tender; season them with salt and fresh herbs, and dinner is ready. You can even start some chicken breasts, burgers, or gourmet sausages under the broiler before adding the

Some Easy Garnishes

Herbs: One of our favorite garnishes is fresh herbs. At our CSA site, we get at least one bunch of fresh herbs with every delivery. Often they are flowering and we snip off the top part of the stem to use for garnish and use the rest to season the dish. Small arrangements of chives, ramps, or trimmed garlic scapes are another easy choice.

Flowers: Because the flowers at most of our CSA sites are organic, we like to use those that are edible for garnishes as well. A sprinkling of edible organic flower petals makes an easy and elegant garnish for salads and desserts. (See page 217 for a list of edible flowers; remember that they must be pesticide-free in order to be used.)

Vegetables: A few clever cuts can turn fresh vegetables into colorful garnishes. Once cut, most should be soaked in ice water at least 30 minutes or as long as overnight until they curl or open up. Here are some classics:

Green Onion Curls or Brushes: Trim the green ends to make the onions the desired length (4 to 6 inches for curls or 1½ to 2 inches for brushes); slice each onion lengthwise starting ½ inch from the root end and extending to the ends of the leaves. Soak.

Radish Flowers: For roses, make 2 rows of angular cuts into the side of each radish. Cut a fine crosshatch into the top center. For bachelor's buttons, cut a crosshatch through the entire radish to within ¼ inch of the stem end. Soak.

vegetables for a meat and vegetable meal. The quick start-up time of broiling is a plus, but you might miss the smoky flavor you get with grilling.

DEEP-FRYING: Who can resist the flavor of deep-fried anything? In the case of vegetables, the technique has unlimited possibilities. Because the vegetables are submerged in the intensely hot oil or melted fat, their flavor and juiciness are trapped by their crisp outer coating, just waiting to be released with the first bite. Although French fries are the quintessential deep-fried vegetable, other options include sweet potato and squash slices or fries;

Tomato Roses: For each rose, cut a thin slice almost through the stem end of a small tomato. When close to the skin on the side opposite your starting point, angle the knife and peel around and around the tomato, removing the skin in a long spiral. Roll up the spiral and stand it on the original slice, flaring the spiral at the top.

Chrysanthemums: For each flower, trim the stem end of a turnip, a rutabaga, an onion, or a 2-inch portion of a large carrot so that it is level. Set the vegetable on its level surface and cut a crosshatch down to within 1/2 inch of the bottom. Soak.

Carrot Curls or Daisies: Peel the carrots. For curls, use the vegetable peeler to cut as many paper-thin lengthwise slices as possible from each carrot. Roll up the slices and fasten them with toothpicks. Soak and remove the toothpicks. For daisies, cut 5 lengthwise furrows into each carrot, slice crosswise, and use or soak.

Leaves: Cut ovals from a green bell pepper with cookie cutters or a knife, use halved and seeded jalapeño peppers, or quarter a small green bell pepper and make lengthwise cuts starting 1/2 inch from the smallest end.

Fruit: Clusters of organic berries, currants, and grapes can be used to garnish any part of a meal; halves of stone fruit can be brushed with a little lemon juice and filled with goat cheese, salsa, chutney, pesto, or anything that goes with the dish; and citrus slices and wedges can be dusted with chopped herbs to accompany seafood and poultry.

batter-coated broccoli, cauliflower, green beans, and peppers; onion chrysanthemums or loaves; fritters of all kinds; and crispy parsley and other greens used as entrée garnishes and toppings.

Deep-frying is easiest in a temperature-controlled fryer, but you can also successfully use a heavy saucepan and a deep-fat thermometer. Because oils and fats are expensive, it is a good idea to select the smallest pan size that will allow you to fry the amount of vegetables you need in several batches. Even though lard gives fried foods a wonderful old-fashioned flavor, it is not easy to find, and most people opt for the easily available vegetable oils. You can use any vegetable oil you have on hand, but if you don't mind the slightly higher cost of peanut or olive oil, either will provide superior flavor to your fried vegetables. Because they will cook quickly, most deep-fried vegetables are cooked at between 360° and 375°F. And if the temperature is maintained properly, the vegetables will be crisp and delicious without taking in the oil. Because high heat does cause molecular changes in the oils and fats available for home use, they should not be reused. Set the pan aside until the oil or fat has come to room temperature, transfer it to a container with a tight-fitting lid, and then dispose of it.

If not using a temperature-controlled fryer, for safety's sake, always deep-fry in a heavy saucepan securely placed on a level burner. Don't fill the pan more than halfway with oil or fat. Heat the oil to the desired temperature slowly. Check the temperature frequently, and be sure to have a slotted spatula, a slotted spoon, or tongs ready to remove the vegetables to paper towels to drain. If the oil should flame, turn off all the burners on the stove, cover the pan with a lid, and sprinkle salt or baking soda over any oil that has spilled from the pan. We're sure this will never happen; we just had to tell you what to do in case, so go ahead and enjoy those fries.

GRILLING: Pre-Columbian inhabitants of this hemisphere were enjoying grilled foods well before European explorers took note, and there is still nothing as enticing as the aroma of dinner cooking on the grill. Grilled vegetables are simply delicious and so easy to do. Quick-cooking ones such as asparagus, corn, eggplant, onions, peppers, summer squash, tomatoes, and zucchini can just be brushed with oil and arranged on a preheated metal grate set about 4 inches above glowing charcoal or hardwood or a gas flame. Vegetables that normally take more than 6 to 8 minutes to cook in boiling water (such as potatoes, sweet potatoes, carrots, and globe and Jerusalem artichokes) should be parboiled (see Parboiling and Blanching, pages 12–13) until almost tender before grilling. Small items such as brussels sprouts, mushrooms, baby squash, and sugar snap peas should be threaded onto metal or well-soaked bamboo skewers before grilling to keep them from slipping through the grate. Long, thin vegetables such as asparagus are much easier to handle if two skewers are inserted, about 2 inches apart, through 4 to 6 pieces.

If using charcoal, we recommend selecting the most natural product you can find and starting the fire with an electric starter or a charcoal chimney. For the sake of your health, the flavor of your grilled organic vegetables, and the environment, avoid chemical starters and charcoal that contains them. Because lighting and monitoring the fire is the most time-consuming part of the process, and grilling the vegetables takes only a few minutes, we like to plan ahead and grill some for the next day as well. The already prepared and chilled grilled vegetables will make great sandwiches, salads, appetizers, or side dishes. Grilling has always been a year-round habit in the warmer half of the country, but now folks are bundling up, brushing the snow from the grill, and enjoying grilled food in the middle of the winter in areas where the food was once housebound for six months of the year. In our area, CSA deliveries continue until the week of Thanksgiving, and we can't think of anything more appropriate than grilled vegetables for Thanksgiving dinner.

MICROWAVING: In a microwave oven, food is cooked by electromagnetic waves that cause the food's water molecules to oscillate around their axes and produce heat. Because the waves penetrate only about 1 inch from the surface of the food, the center of microwaved food must be cooked by heat transferred from its outer edge. Microwaves can pass through glass and ceramic containers but are deflected by metal ones. Vegetables are actually one of the things microwave ovens do well because most vegetables don't need long cooking, don't have the density that is a problem with larger items, and don't require surface browning to develop flavor.

Microwaving cooks vegetables quickly, right in their serving container, without excessive nutrient or color loss, and with little cleanup necessary. In addition to the "don't microwave in metal" rule, here are some other things to keep in mind when microwaving: Select a microwave with a turntable to avoid having to turn foods several times during cooking. Covering foods will add steam to the process, and vegetables will cook faster and more evenly. Vegetables microwave more evenly in a round container because the waves all aim toward the center rather than toward another side. Arrange the densest part of the vegetables toward the outside of the container so they receive the initial microwaves and pass along their heat to the parts that require less cooking. While one or two servings microwave very quickly, larger numbers of servings increase the cooking time, eventually reaching the point where it would be faster to use another cooking method. Microwaves increase the flavor released by herbs and spices, so you might want to reduce the amount used or add them at the end of the cooking time. Remove vegetables from the microwave when they are almost tender because they will continue to cook internally for several minutes at room temperature.

PANFRYING OR SAUTÉING: Panfrying means cooking in a skillet (or frying pan) over medium to high heat with just enough oil or melted fat to slightly come up the sides of whatever is being fried, not cover it. It provides the crisp exterior and decadent flavor of deep-frying, but the vegetables will experience a bit more moisture loss because the top surface is exposed during the first half of cooking. Frying is quick, uses less oil or fat than deep-frying, and requires little cleanup. Sautéing is almost the same as frying except that it uses only enough oil or fat to glaze the surface of the skillet and keep the vegetables from sticking. The two terms seem to be used interchangeably these days, and, in truth, with many people reducing the amount of oil and fat in their recipes, most of our frying is now sautéing.

Whatever you call it, this is a fast and flavorful way to prepare breaded vegetables such as fried green tomatoes or fried squash; vegetable cakes, pancakes, or "burgers"; potato, sweet potato, or mixed-vegetable "home fries"; Italian-style stuffed peppers or stuffed zucchini blossoms; and any vegetable you want to serve seared and crisp-tender. If you are sautéing chopped or sliced vegetables, you can toss them rather than stirring them to keep them from sticking in the skillet.

PARBOILING AND BLANCHING: Separated only by time, parboiling and blanching are so close in definition that we are going to explain them together. To do either, heat a pot of water to boiling, add the vegetables for the prescribed amount of time, drain the vegetables, and plunge them into ice water to stop the cooking. If the recipe calls for blanching, drain the vegetables immediately after their plunge into the boiling water. This will loosen the skins of tomatoes and fruit for easy peeling, set the color and flavor of vegetables such as broccoli for crudités and green peas for canning or freezing, stop the enzymatic browning on the surface of sliced vegetables and fruit, and reduce the volume of greens in order to add them to a recipe.

When a recipe calls for parboiling, it should give a time or a desired end point so you will know how long to boil the vegetables before draining them. It will achieve everything that blanching does and in addition will start tenderizing the vegetables so that they can be grilled or broiled quickly, added to faster-cooking foods in a stir-fry, or layered with a sauce in a gratin that doesn't take hours to finish. Parboiling and blanching are pretreatments that make life easier for a busy cook.

POACHING: No, this has nothing to do with stopping along the road and snatching a few ears of corn from a field—farmers hate that and usually plant the sweet corn where you can't find it anyway. Poaching is gently cooking fruits or vegetables in a liquid that is barely simmering—just below the boiling point. The liquid can be sugar syrup, fruit juice, wine, seasoned water, meat or vegetable stock, or any other flavorful liquid. This is especially good for fragile foods such as peaches, pears, berries, baby summer squash, French green beans, and our Spinach Gnocchi (pages 196–97). Once cooked, the food is carefully removed to the serving dish using a slotted spoon. Then you can turn up the heat and reduce all or part of the poaching liquid to use for a sauce.

PRESSURE-COOKING: When you heat water in an open saucepan at sea level, it boils at 212°F and starts to escape into the air as steam. In the securely closed atmosphere of a pressure cooker, the steam can't escape and pushes down on the hot water, preventing it from boiling at the usual 212°F, so the water continues to heat and produce hotter and hotter steam in an effort to come to a boil. When vegetables are prepared in a pressure cooker, they are placed on a rack above the water and the pressure is usually set at 15 pounds. At that setting, the vegetables are cooking in steam that has been superheated to 250°F. As you can guess, this method greatly reduces cooking time, but, to avoid overcooking, it should be reserved for vegetables that would need to boil 10 or more minutes without the increased pressure to become tender. It is a big help with end-of-the-season beets and rutabagas, but broccoli or asparagus would be overcooked before the pan had reached full pressure.

ROASTING: Once called baked, as in "baked potatoes," roasted vegetables are "hot!" And there is nothing easier. You simply toss the prepared vegetables in olive oil and seasonings, spread them on an aluminum foil–covered (makes it easier to clean up) tray, and roast them until they are crisp-tender. The initial heat on the surface of the vegetables seals in the moisture, and the vegetables brown on the outside as they become tender and juicy on the inside. The only secret is that different vegetables achieve perfection at different times; so when you see a tray of perfectly roasted mixed vegetables come from the wood oven of a restaurant, they were roasted separately until almost done and then mixed together for the final few minutes. Do the same thing at home and you will always be successful. Many of the things you might do on a grill, such as corn in the husk, wedges of baking potatoes, and split zucchini, can be just as successfully roasted.

STEAMING: Steaming is an excellent way to cook vegetables. Because they are suspended above the boiling liquid, either on a rack or in a special steamer, they come in contact only with condensation from the steam, not with the liquid, and so lose fewer nutrients. Steaming also preserves the color and shape of the vegetables and seals in flavor and moisture. While steaming will take a bit longer than boiling to cook the vegetables to the same degree of doneness, the time saved in bringing the smaller amount of liquid to a boil may compensate for that difference. Excellent multilevel steamers allow you to prepare a whole meal at once with only one piece of equipment to clean up.

STIR-FRYING OR PANNING: In this technique, vegetables cook in the small amount of moisture clinging to their leaves or in the moisture that escapes from their cut surfaces. A very small amount of oil or fat is heated in a heavy skillet or wok, and sliced, shredded, or chopped vegetables are added. The mixture is cooked over fairly high heat, stirring constantly, until the vegetables are crisp-tender. Sometimes a sauce is added at the end or the pan is covered and the heat reduced to preserve the natural vegetable juices. This method is quick, retains the color, flavor, and texture of the vegetables, and produces a whole meal in one pan.

What Is Crisp-Tender?

Throughout this book, you will find that recipes tell you to cook vegetables until crisp-tender. Until the last ten years or so, the prevailing concept of vegetable cooking was to cook vegetables a long time, often an hour, until they were very soft and had lost most of their color and flavor. These days, more and more people are cooking vegetables just to the point where the tip of a sharp knife will pierce the vegetable without trouble, but it still has a little crunch—the vegetable equivalent of al dente pasta. This is crisp-tender, or, as some people say, tender-crisp, and vegetables cooked to this stage retain their shape, color, texture, and, most of all, flavor.

Preserving Vegetables

CANNING: The first modern development in food preservation, canning was introduced in 1809 by Nicolas Appert, after fourteen years of experimentation in response to a prize offered in 1795 by Napoléon for a method of preserving foods for troops on the battlefield. Appert was awarded the prize in 1810. The process entails vacuum-sealing foods in glass containers that are then heated to high temperatures to keep out oxygen and to destroy the organisms that produce spoilage. At first, canning was done by a boiling-water-bath method, which heated the foods to a temperature of 212°F for a prescribed period of time. A few decades later, pressure-canning was developed, making it possible to heat foods as high as 265°F; this is a much safer process for nonacid vegetables and meats. These are still the two choices of canning methods. High-acid and high-sugar foods can be sealed using the water-bath method, while low-acid vegetables must be canned in a pressure canner.

Commercially canned foods were popularized in the United States during the Civil War; home canning increased in popularity during World War I and the Depression and reached its peak during World War II. Today, canning has taken on a different role in the preservation of the summer harvest. Offering the advantage of room-temperature storage, canning is still the preferred processing for pickles, relishes, jams, jellies, tomato products, and some fruits. Because of the amount of work associated with this technique, today's home canners look for value added in the end product. They like to produce items that make good gifts and are ready to use when opened, such as salsa, tomato sauce, jams, jellies, and pickles. We have included only a few recipes that call for canning the item after it is prepared and those provide the directions for doing so.

DRYING OR DEHYDRATION: Drying is the most ancient technique for preserving foods. Although in the past it might have been done using just the power of the sun, that is not really practical in most of the United States. In order to dehydrate foods before they have a chance to spoil, both high temperature and low humidity must be maintained for a long period of time.

If you are interested in drying foods, an electric dehydrator is a good investment. Tomatoes, onions, corn, beans, apples, peaches, and berries can be dried at the peak of their season, stored in sealed jars, and used all year round. It is as easy as selecting high-quality produce, pretreating it, and arranging it on the dehydrator trays. Pretreating includes rinsing, peeling, slicing, and dipping in lemon juice or another antioxidant, if necessary. Drying time is dependent upon the natural water content of the product, the size and thickness of the pieces, the humidity in the air, and the power of your dehydrator. When the fruit or vegetable has reached the right degree of dehydration, pack it in a clean, airtight container (such as a canning jar) and store in a cool, dry area. Degree of dehydration varies for different foods and different purposes—corn is usually dried until crisp, as are the paper-thin fruit and vegetable garnishes used by chefs today, while tomatoes and some fruit are often dried until leathery but not brittle. The recipe, a preserving guide, or the information that comes with the dehydrator will help you decide how much moisture you want to remove. The more moisture you remove, the longer the product may be kept.

FREEZING: Freezing is probably the best choice when, at the end of the summer, the share of produce that CSA members receive becomes more than they can use in four or five days. Freezing preserves the flavor, color, and nutritive value of the foods; it requires little equipment and even less time; and it is so easy that you can package and freeze one container or many in a few minutes after dinner. Because freezing does not kill bacteria, yeasts, or mold

Some General Hints for Cooking Vegetables

- Never add baking soda to the cooking water; it makes the vegetables mushy and destroys vitamins.
- If you're cooking a red or purple vegetable, add a slice of apple or some lemon juice to the water to keep its color bright.
- Don't try to reheat cooked vegetables in water. They will turn gray and mushy. Heat them in the microwave or in a sauce.
- Green vegetables will not lose their color as fast if cooked without a lid.

and doesn't deactivate enzymes (it just slows them all down), it is best to cook vegetables as you would to serve them. Let them cool quickly to room temperature, and package them in airtight, moistureproof containers. To prevent freezer burn, which is caused by the circulation of air in the freezer, it is essential that all surfaces of the food be covered with freezer-safe packaging so they don't come in contact with the air. Be sure to label and date the packages, then freeze and store them at 0°F to prevent the development of large ice crystals within the food.

PICKLING AND JELLY-MAKING: Pickling is another ancient method of preserving foods. Vegetables (and sometimes fruit) are packed in either a salt-water brine or a spicy sugar-and-vinegar solution and chilled for short-term use or vacuum-packed for long-term, room-temperature storage. The recipe can be as simple as combining chopped vegetables with vinegar and sugar for a refrigerated relish or as time-consuming as a favorite watermelon pickle recipe that is drained, then covered with freshly boiled syrup every morning for three to five days, depending on the version. We have included just a few simple ones that may be processed for long-term storage or not, and all the directions are provided.

Homemade jams and jellies are remarkably easy to make and are not only perfect spreads for breads but are often the secret ingredient in sauces, salad dressings, ice cream toppings, glazes, and desserts. At the height of the season, many CSA groups will let you preorder extra fruit and vegetables for jelly-making and canning. Nothing compares to homemade jams and jellies prepared from freshly harvested, naturally ripened, organic fruit.

Here's what you can do with some of the most common vegetables from CSA farms:

VEGETABLE	SERVE RAW	BOIL	BRAISE	BROIL	DEEP-FRY	FRY	GRILL	MICROWAVE	PARBOIL*	POACH	PRESSURE	ROAST	SAUTÉ	STEAM	STIR-FRY	CAN/PICKLE	DRY	FREEZE
Artichoke, Globe		x	x	x			x	x	x			x	x	x		x		x
Artichoke, Jerusalem	x	x	x	x		x	x	x	x			x	x	x	x			
Asparagus		x		x	x		x	x		x		x		x	x			x
Beans, Dried		x	x					x				x						x
Beans, Fresh		x			x	x	x			x			x	x	x	x	x	x
Beet Greens		x	x			x	x	x	x				x	x	x			x
Beets	x	x	x	x			x	x	x		x	x		x		x		x
Broccoli	x	x			x		x	x					x	x				x
Brussels Sprouts		x	x	x			x	x	x	x	x	x	x	x				x
Cabbage	x	x	x					x	x	x	x		x	x	x			x
Carrots	x	x	x	x		x	x	x	x		x	x	x	x	x	x		x
Cauliflower	x	x	x		x		x	x	x	x	x	x	x	x	x			x
Celeriac	x	x	x					x	x	x	x	x	x	x				
Celery	x	x	x					x		x	x		x	x				
Chicory	x	x	x					x			x		x	x				x
Collards		x	x					x	x	x	x		x	x	x			x
Corn	x	x		x			x	x				x		x	x	x	x	x
Cucumbers	x															x		
Eggplant				x	x	x	x					x	x		x			
Endive, Belgian	x		x	x			x	x		x			x	x				x
Endive, Curly	x	x	x					x			x		x	x				x
Escarole	x	x	x					x		x	x		x	x	x			x
Fennel	x	x	x	x		x	x	x	x	x	x	x	x	x	x			
Garlic	x	x	x	x	x	x	x		x			x	x		x			
Green Onions	x	x	x	x	x	x	x		x				x	x	x			x

VEGETABLE	SERVE RAW	BOIL	BRAISE	BROIL	DEEP-FRY	FRY	GRILL	MICROWAVE	PARBOIL*	POACH	PRESSURE	ROAST	SAUTÉ	STEAM	STIR-FRY	CAN/PICKLE	DRY	FREEZE
Kale		x	x					x	x	x	x			x	x	x		x
Kohlrabi		x	x					x	x	x	x	x		x	x			
Leeks		x	x	x	x	x	x	x	x	x	x	x	x	x	x			x
Lettuce	x													x				
Mustard		x	x					x	x	x	x			x	x	x		
Okra		x		x	x	x	x	x					x	x				x
Onions	x	x	x	x	x	x	x	x	x	x	x	x	x	x	x	x	x	x
Parsnips		x	x		x	x	x	x	x	x	x	x	x	x				
Peas	x	x								x				x	x		x	x
Peppers	x			x	x	x	x	x					x	x	x	x	x	x
Potatoes		x	x	x	x	x	x	x	x	x	x	x	x		x			
Pumpkin		x									x	x		x				x
Radishes	x	x	x							x		x		x	x			
Rutabagas		x	x						x		x	x		x				x
Salsify		x	x					x	x	x	x			x		x		x
Sorrel		x	x					x	x	x	x			x		x		x
Spinach	x	x	x					x	x	x	x			x	x			x
Squash, Summer	x	x		x	x	x	x	x	x				x	x	x	x	x	x
Squash, Winter		x	x					x	x	x	x			x				x
Sweet Potatoes		x	x					x	x	x	x			x				x
Swiss Chard		x	x					x	x	x	x			x		x		x
Tomatoes	x	x				x	x						x			x		
Turnip Greens		x	x					x	x	x	x			x	x	x		x
Turnips		x	x						x		x	x		x				x

*The vegetables we have selected are parboiled to reduce their volume or cooking time. They should then be drained and cooked by another method, often with other quick-cooking vegetables, before serving.

CHAPTER TWO

BASIC RECIPES

BASIC VEGETABLE QUICHE

MAKES 6 SERVINGS

From Swiss chard season (early summer) to winter squash season (late fall), this is always a hit at our potlucks. We have included two easy pastry recipes and have tested this quiche with homemade pastry in standard 9-inch glass and enamel pie plates.

Pastry for 1 (9-inch) single-crust pie
  (recipes follow)
4 bacon slices or 2 tablespoons olive oil
1 cup chopped green or yellow onions
3 cups prepared vegetables (see Note)
3 tablespoons all-purpose flour
½ teaspoon salt

¼ teaspoon dried thyme
⅛ teaspoon freshly milled black
  pepper
2 large eggs
1 cup half-and-half or whole milk
1½ cups grated Jarlsberg, Swiss,
  or your favorite cheese

Prepare the piecrust. On a floured board, roll out the pastry to make an 11-inch round; fit into a standard 9-inch pie pan. Fold over the edge of the dough on the pan rim and flute.

Preheat the oven to 375°F. Sauté the bacon in a large skillet over medium heat until crisp; remove to paper towels to drain. Reserve 2 tablespoons of the drippings in the skillet. (If not using bacon, heat the oil in a large skillet over medium heat.) Add the onions and sauté until lightly browned, about 3 minutes. Stir in the prepared vegetables and cook until heated through, 2 to 3 minutes. Stir in the flour, ½ teaspoon salt (use ¾ teaspoon if not using bacon), the thyme, and the pepper.

Beat the eggs in a medium bowl until frothy; brush a little egg over the bottom of the piecrust. Beat the half-and-half into the remaining eggs. Layer half of the cheese, the vegetable mixture, and the remaining cheese into the piecrust. If using bacon, crumble and sprinkle over the cheese. Pour the cream mixture over all. Bake the quiche for 35 to 40 minutes, until the center appears set when the pie plate is gently tapped. Set aside for 5 minutes before cutting.

NOTE: Almost any vegetable or mixture of vegetables can be used in a quiche. Slice or julienne larger vegetables. If you are using asparagus, broccoli, celery, eggplant, fresh corn, bell peppers, summer squash, mushrooms, or zucchini, they should be added to the skillet raw, and sautéed with the onions. Carrots, green or yellow beans, fresh peas, potatoes, sweet potatoes, and winter squash should be parboiled and drained thoroughly before adding. Greens such as arugula, beet greens, collards, kale, mustard, spinach, Swiss chard, and turnip greens should be steamed, simmered, or stir-fried until wilted, thoroughly drained, and coarsely chopped before adding.

Plain Pastry

MAKES ENOUGH FOR
1 (9-INCH) PIECRUST

1 ½ cups all-purpose flour
¼ teaspoon salt

8 tablespoons (1 stick) cold unsalted butter

Combine the flour and salt in a medium bowl. Cut in the butter with a pastry blender or two knives until the mixture resembles coarse crumbs.

Sprinkle 4 to 6 tablespoons cold water over the flour a little at a time and stir with a fork until the pastry forms a ball when lightly pressed. Flatten the dough, wrap, and chill for at least 30 minutes.

Easy Whole Wheat Pastry

MAKES ENOUGH FOR
1 (9-INCH) PIECRUST

1 cup whole wheat flour
½ cup unsifted all-purpose flour

¼ teaspoon salt
½ cup vegetable shortening

Combine the flours and salt in a medium bowl. Cut in the shortening with a pastry blender or two knives until the mixture resembles coarse crumbs. Sprinkle 4 to 5 tablespoons cold water over the flour a little at a time and stir with a fork until the pastry forms a ball when lightly pressed. Flatten the dough, wrap, and chill for at least 30 minutes.

BASIC SOUFFLÉ

The secret to a perfect soufflé is using fresh eggs and gently incorporating the beaten egg whites with the vegetable-puree mixture. You can use asparagus, beets, broccoli, carrots, cauliflower, peas, pumpkin, summer or winter squash, and greens such as chard, mustard, and spinach. (See Basic Purees, page 30).

¾ cup vegetable puree
6 large eggs
4 tablespoons (½ stick) unsalted butter
¼ cup very finely chopped onion
3 tablespoons all-purpose flour
¾ teaspoon salt

1 teaspoon chopped fresh dill, marjoram, oregano, or thyme (see page 215)
⅛ teaspoon freshly milled black pepper
1¼ cups milk
4 tablespoons grated Parmigiano-Reggiano cheese

Prepare the vegetable puree. Separate the eggs, placing the whites in a large bowl and the yolks in a small bowl. Gradually beat the puree into the yolks with a wire whisk.

Melt the butter in a medium skillet. Add the onion and sauté until tender, about 3 minutes. Stir in the flour, the salt, your choice of herb, and the pepper; gradually stir in the milk. Bring the mixture to a boil over medium heat, stirring constantly until smooth and thickened. Fold the puree mixture into the thickened sauce along with 3 tablespoons of the cheese. Let cool to room temperature.

Preheat the oven to 350°F. Measure and cut a 26-inch-long piece of wax paper. Fold the paper in thirds lengthwise. Lightly grease one side. Fit the paper, greased side in, around the outside of a 1½-quart soufflé dish with at least 2 inches above the top of the dish. Tie tightly with string.

With an electric mixer on high speed, beat the whites until stiff peaks form. Gently fold some of the whites into the vegetable mixture. Then fold the mixture into the remaining beaten whites. Gently spoon the mixture into the prepared soufflé dish. Sprinkle with the remaining 1 tablespoon cheese.

Bake the soufflé for 40 to 45 minutes, until the top is golden brown and the center does not shake when the dish is gently tapped. Serve immediately.

There is nothing faster than an omelet for breakfast, lunch, or dinner when you are serving a small number of people. This recipe serves one but can be multiplied to serve more. We suggest using an 8- to 9-inch pan for a double recipe and a 10-inch pan for four. If serving more than that, you might want to go to a second pan or cook the omelets one at a time and keep them warm in a very low temperature oven.

2 large eggs
1 tablespoon milk, water, stock, or sour
   cream
1/8 teaspoon salt

1/8 teaspoon freshly milled black pepper
2 teaspoons vegetable oil or unsalted
   butter
1/2 cup warm omelet filling (see below)

Whisk together the eggs, milk, salt, and pepper. Heat the oil in a 7- or 8-inch omelet pan or heavy skillet over medium-high heat.

Pour in the egg mixture, tilting the pan to distribute the egg evenly. As the egg sets, push it toward the center of the pan with an inverted spatula and swirl the uncooked egg onto the pan surface. When the top surface has just set, fill, fold in half, and slide onto a serving plate.

OMELET FILLINGS: To fill one single-serving omelet, combine about 1/2 cup of any hot cooked chopped or thinly sliced vegetable or mixture of vegetables with 3 tablespoons grated American, blue, Cheddar, Monterey Jack, Muenster, or mozzarella cheese (or 1 tablespoon Parmesan); salt and freshly milled black pepper to taste; and 1/8 teaspoon dried basil, marjoram, oregano, rosemary, or thyme. Cooked meat, poultry, or fish can make up part of the 1/2 cup filling as well.

BASIC OMELETS AND FRITTATAS

Omelet

MAKES 1 SERVING

Frittata

MAKES 4 SERVINGS

This Italian-style omelet couldn't be easier. Any cooked vegetable can be used and you can serve the frittata right from the pan. Mix and match the cheese and herbs with the vegetables you have chosen.

2 tablespoons olive oil
1 medium onion, thinly sliced
1 garlic clove, finely chopped
2 cups cooked chopped or thinly sliced
   vegetables
6 large eggs
½ teaspoon salt
⅛ teaspoon freshly milled black
   pepper

¼ cup grated Cheddar, Muenster,
   or Swiss cheese
2 tablespoons grated Parmigiano-
   Reggiano cheese
¼ to ½ teaspoon dried basil,
   marjoram, oregano, rosemary,
   or thyme (optional)

Heat 1 tablespoon of the oil in a heavy 10-inch skillet with a broilerproof handle over medium heat. Add the onion and garlic and sauté until just tender, about 3 minutes. Add the vegetables and cook, stirring, until hot.

Meanwhile, whisk together the eggs, salt, and pepper in a medium bowl; fold in the hot vegetable mixture, the cheeses, and the herb, if using. Heat the remaining 1 tablespoon oil in the same skillet over very low heat. Pour in the egg-and-vegetable mixture, spreading with a spatula to distribute evenly. Cook, covered, until the top surface has just set, 8 to 10 minutes.

Preheat the broiler halfway through the cooking time. Broil the frittata just until the top surface browns. Cut into 4 wedges and serve.

The only thing that makes a casserole a gratin is the crisp, well-browned, broiled topping. You can use buttered bread crumbs, grated cheese, a mixture of the two, or nothing at all over layers of cooked vegetables.

1 pound potatoes, turnips, rutabagas, sweet potatoes, or Jerusalem artichokes, peeled and thinly sliced
1 pound leafy greens, cabbage, zucchini, summer squash, fennel, Belgian endive, or cauliflower, rinsed and drained, if necessary, and thinly sliced, or an additional pound of roots and tubers above
4 tablespoons olive oil or unsalted butter

1 large onion, chopped
2 garlic cloves, finely chopped (optional)
2 cups milk, stock, or cooled vegetable cooking liquid
1/4 cup all-purpose flour
Salt and freshly milled black pepper
1 1/4 cups grated Cheddar, Swiss, Muenster, Monterey Jack, or other cheese
1/2 cup fresh bread crumbs or panko (Japanese bread crumbs)

Cook the root vegetables in boiling salted water for 5 to 7 minutes, until the surface starts to look cooked. Drain; save the cooking liquid and let cool to use for the sauce, if desired. Blanch the pound of more tender vegetables; drain thoroughly.

Preheat the oven to 375°F. Lightly grease a 2-quart gratin or shallow baking dish.

Heat 2 tablespoons of the oil in a skillet over medium heat. Sauté the onion and garlic, if using, until they start to brown, about 4 minutes.

Whisk the milk into the flour in a small bowl. Whisk the milk mixture into the onion mixture and cook, stirring constantly, until the sauce is bubbly and thickened. Add salt and pepper to taste.

Layer half of the root vegetables, 1/3 cup sauce, 1/4 cup cheese, half of the tender vegetables, 1/3 cup sauce, and 1/4 cup cheese. Repeat, ending with 1 cup sauce and 1/2 cup cheese. Combine the bread crumbs and the remaining 2 tablespoons oil. If using butter, melt the remaining 2 tablespoons before combining. Sprinkle crumbs over the cheese.

Bake for 35 to 40 minutes, until the root vegetables are tender and the top is well browned.

BASIC CREPES

MAKES 6 SERVINGS

We can't think of anything that chives don't go with, but if you would like to use another fresh herb instead, or add it in addition, why not? If you leave out the chives or other herb and add a little sugar, this recipe makes excellent sweet crepes. Fill them with about 4 cups of fresh berries and some sweetened whipped cream instead of vegetables and cheese, and you've got dessert.

¾ cup all-purpose flour
¼ teaspoon salt
2 large eggs
1 cup milk
1 teaspoon finely chopped fresh chives

2 tablespoons vegetable oil
6 cups seasoned cooked vegetables
¼ cup grated Gruyère, Muenster,
    or Monterey Jack cheese

Combine the flour and salt in a medium bowl. Beat in the eggs and milk until the mixture is almost smooth. Strain the mixture into a measuring cup or small pitcher and stir in the chives.

Heat a crepe pan or heavy 8-inch skillet over medium heat; brush the bottom with some of the oil. Ladle about ⅓ cup batter into the skillet; tip the pan to cover the bottom with batter and create a 6-inch round crepe. Cook the crepe until the top is set and the bottom is lightly browned, about 2 minutes. Carefully turn the crepe and cook the other side briefly. Remove the finished crepe to a sheet of wax paper. Repeat to make 11 more.

Preheat the oven to 350°F. Combine the vegetables and cheese. Spread the crepes out on a work surface. Divide the filling among the crepes. Fold the crepes in quarters and stand them up in a baking dish or roll them around the filling and arrange in the baking dish. Bake until warm and the tops of the crepes are crisp, about 15 minutes.

Stock is the secret ingredient of any restaurant kitchen. This simple recipe will help you make it at home. And once it is made, you can quickly turn it into either a clear or a cream soup. You will notice lots of optional ingredients listed; they will give the stock more flavor but may not be suitable for the soups or sauces you will be making. Decide how you will use the stock and select flavors that are compatible.

BASIC STOCK AND SOUPS

2 tablespoons olive oil
1 large onion or 6 green onions,
  coarsely chopped
2 celery stalks, coarsely chopped
2 medium carrots, coarsely chopped
3 parsley sprigs
4 garlic cloves, sliced
1 sprig fresh thyme or basil
4 ounces white mushrooms, coarsely
  chopped (optional)

1 large green bell pepper, coarsely
  chopped (optional)
Bones from 1 roasting chicken, bones
  from 1 beef rib roast, or 2 beef soup
  bones (optional)
1 large tomato, coarsely chopped
  (optional)
Salt and freshly milled black pepper

Heat the oil in a heavy 4-quart saucepan over medium heat. Add the onion, celery, carrots, parsley, garlic, and thyme. If using the mushrooms or bell pepper, add here as well. Cook, stirring, until the vegetables begin to brown, about 5 minutes. Add 3 quarts water, the chicken or beef bones, if using, and the tomato, if using. Bring to a boil over high heat; reduce the heat to low and cook, uncovered, until reduced by half, about 30 minutes.

Strain the mixture into a clean saucepan or bowl, pressing the ingredients to remove all the stock. Add salt and black pepper to taste. Use the stock to make soup or let cool to room temperature and freeze in 1-cup containers to use in sauces.

CLEAR SOUPS: Soups make a satisfying lunch or supper with not much trouble or cleanup. You can mix and match the produce from your CSA share to make a different soup every week. For 6 servings, simmer 3 to 6 cups of chopped or julienned vegetables in 6 cups homemade stock or low-sodium canned broth until just tender. If using mixed vegetables, be sure to add less-tender vegetables (such as beets, carrots, Jerusalem artichokes, lima beans, parsnips, potatoes, sweet potatoes, turnips, and winter squash) first, moderately tender vegetables (such as brussels sprouts, cabbage, chard, collards, escarole, green beans, fresh peas, and kale) about 7 to 10 minutes later, and quick-cooking vegetables (such as lettuce, snow and sugar snap peas, spinach, and fresh herbs) for the last 3 to 5 minutes. If using dried beans, parboil the beans until almost tender before adding. Fully cooked meat or poultry or uncooked seafood can be added for the last 5 minutes.

CREAM SOUPS: An elegant first course for a holiday or company dinner, cream soups can be made a day ahead and are ready in the refrigerator to be served cold or gently reheated depending upon the season. For 6 servings, combine 4 cups homemade stock or low-sodium canned broth and 2 cups vegetable puree (see page 30). Garnish with a swirl of sour cream or some chopped fresh herbs.

CLASSIC SAUCES

Many classic sauces that are delicious on vegetables are based on raw eggs. But don't let the recent concern about food safety make you give them up. The following recipes, adapted from ones created by the American Egg Board, heat the sauce mixtures just to boiling, destroying the bacteria that have caused the concern. It is still important to keep the sauces well chilled and to use them within two days.

Mayonnaise

MAKES 1 CUP

2 large egg yolks
3 tablespoons white wine vinegar
   or lemon juice
1 1/2 teaspoons sugar

1/2 teaspoon dry mustard
1/4 teaspoon salt
1/8 teaspoon freshly milled black pepper
3/4 cup vegetable oil

Combine the egg yolks, the vinegar, 1 tablespoon water, the sugar, the mustard, the salt, and the pepper in a small saucepan. Cook over very low heat, stirring constantly, just until the mixture begins to bubble. Transfer to a blender and set aside for 5 minutes.

Cover and blend at high speed, very gradually adding the oil through the opening in the lid until all the oil has been incorporated and the mixture is thick. Transfer to a storage container and refrigerate; use within 2 days.

3 large egg yolks
3 tablespoons lemon juice
8 tablespoons (1 stick) unsalted butter,
  thinly sliced

Salt
⅛ teaspoon paprika
⅛ teaspoon ground red pepper

Combine the egg yolks, the lemon juice, and 3 tablespoons water in a small saucepan. Cook over very low heat, stirring constantly, just until the mixture begins to bubble. Stir in the butter, a few slices at a time, until all the butter has been incorporated and the mixture is thick. Fold in salt to taste and the paprika and red pepper. Spoon over cooked vegetables or meats and serve, or transfer to a storage container and refrigerate. If chilled, warm very gently before serving and use within 2 days.

BÉARNAISE SAUCE: Gently simmer ¼ cup white wine, 1 tablespoon tarragon vinegar or white wine vinegar, 1 tablespoon finely chopped shallot or onion, and ¾ teaspoon dried tarragon until most of the liquid has evaporated. Fold the hot mixture into the prepared ¾ cup Hollandaise Sauce and use as directed above.

BASIC PUREES

MAKES 1 CUP

Purees are colorful and comforting as a side dish (we like to pair two compatible flavors and swirl them in the serving bowl) and are an essential first step to vegetable soufflés, cream soups, and breads. Because they are simply made from fully cooked vegetables and seasonings, you really need to know only how much to cook and how long.

1 pound vegetables, rinsed or peeled and cut into 1-inch chunks, if necessary

½ teaspoon chopped fresh thyme, oregano, basil, cilantro, or rosemary, or ⅛ teaspoon dried (optional)
Salt and freshly milled black pepper (optional)

Combine the vegetables, water to cover, and the herb, if using, in a small saucepan. Heat to boiling over high heat; reduce the heat and cook, covered, until tender.

Drain the vegetables thoroughly, reserving the cooking liquid. Puree the vegetables in a food processor or blender, adding the cooking liquid 1 tablespoon at a time until the mixture is smooth and creamy yet stiff enough to maintain a furrow when a spoon is pulled through the mixture. Add salt and pepper to taste.

Use the puree as directed in the recipe of your choice, or prepare the puree recipe in multiples and serve as a side dish, allowing about ¾ cup puree per serving.

BASIC TOMATO SAUCES

Traditional Tomato Sauce

MAKES 4 SERVINGS

When the tomatoes are so ripe that you can smell the sauce as they come off the truck, hurry home and make several batches of this slow-cooked sauce for the freezer.

1 tablespoon olive oil
1 large onion, thinly sliced
1 large green bell pepper, chopped
2 garlic cloves, finely chopped
2 pounds ripe plum tomatoes, skinned (see page 32) and quartered

1 cup dry white or red wine
1 tablespoon coarsely chopped fresh basil, or 1 teaspoon dried
1 ½ teaspoons coarsely chopped fresh oregano, or ½ teaspoon dried
Salt and freshly milled black pepper

Heat the oil in a large sauce pot. Add the onion, bell pepper, and garlic and sauté over high heat, stirring until the onion begins to brown, about 4 minutes. Add the tomatoes, wine, basil, and oregano. Bring the mixture to a boil over high heat; reduce the heat to low, cover, and simmer for 1 hour, stirring occasionally. Add salt and pepper to taste and serve.

In a hurry? You can prepare this quick sauce in the time it takes to cook the pasta. But take a moment to savor the flavor of vine-ripened organic tomatoes.

1 tablespoon olive oil
1 large red onion, coarsely chopped
1 large yellow bell pepper, chopped
4 garlic cloves, finely chopped
2 pounds ripe plum tomatoes, skinned
  (see page 32) and coarsely chopped

1 tablespoon coarsely chopped fresh
  basil, or 1 teaspoon dried
1 1/2 teaspoons coarsely chopped fresh
  oregano, or 1/2 teaspoon dried
Salt and freshly milled black pepper

Heat the oil in a large sauce pot. Add the onion, bell pepper, and garlic and sauté over medium heat, stirring until the onion is just tender, about 7 minutes.

Add the tomatoes, basil, and oregano; bring the mixture to a boil and cook just until the tomatoes are heated through, 4 to 5 minutes. Add salt and pepper to taste and serve.

BASIC FRIED VEGETABLES AND FRITTERS

Fried Vegetables

MAKES 4 SERVINGS

Whether you are making fried green tomatoes, fried zucchini, fried eggplant, or any other vegetable that is good breaded, this old-fashioned coating will be delicious.

Sliced vegetables (see Note)
1 large egg
1 tablespoon milk or water
¼ teaspoon salt
⅛ teaspoon freshly milled black
  pepper
1 cup seasoned dried bread crumbs,
  cornmeal, or whole wheat flour,
  or 1 ½ cups fresh bread crumbs,
  panko (Japanese bread crumbs),
  or crushed cornflakes

¾ teaspoon chopped fresh basil, dill,
  marjoram, oregano, or thyme,
  or ¼ teaspoon dried (optional)
2 to 4 tablespoons olive or vegetable
  oil, unsalted butter, or vegetable
  shortening

Parboil and thoroughly drain the vegetables, if necessary. Preheat the oven to 300°F to keep the fried vegetables warm, if desired. Whisk the egg, milk, salt, and pepper in a pie plate. Place the crumbs and herb, if using, in a plastic bag.

Dip several vegetable slices at a time into the egg mixture and then shake in the crumbs until coated. Heat 1 tablespoon of the oil in a large skillet over medium heat. Add as many breaded slices as will fit, and fry until they are

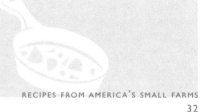

golden on one side, 3 to 5 minutes. Turn the slices, adding more oil as necessary, and cook until tender and brown on the other side, 3 to 5 minutes. Place on a baking sheet and keep warm in the oven. Repeat until all the vegetables have been fried. Season to taste with salt and pepper and serve.

NOTE: For 4 servings, you will need 2 pounds firm tomatoes or green tomatoes, 1½ pounds eggplant or zucchini, or 1½ pounds parboiled sweet onions or sweet potatoes.

Fritters

MAKES 8 FRITTERS

You can use almost any vegetable you have on hand, or mix several, for these no-fuss little cakes.

1½ cups vegetables (see Note)	¼ teaspoon sugar
1 large egg	2 green onions, finely chopped
¼ cup milk	1 teaspoon chopped fresh basil, dill,
¼ cup all-purpose flour	or cilantro
½ teaspoon salt	Vegetable oil

Prepare the vegetables and have them ready to add. Beat the egg until fluffy. Beat in the milk, flour, salt, and sugar. Fold vegetables into the egg mixture with the onions and herb.

Heat 1 tablespoon oil in a large, heavy skillet. Drop generously rounded tablespoons of the batter into the pan and spread to make 2½- to 3-inch rounds. Fry until golden on one side, 3 to 5 minutes. Turn the fritters, add more oil, if necessary, and fry until golden and cooked through, about 4 minutes longer. Serve immediately.

NOTE: You can use any or a mixture of the following vegetables: coarsely shredded carrots, turnips, summer or winter squash, sweet potatoes, or zucchini; fresh corn kernels; chopped broccoli or cauliflower; or thinly sliced cabbage, chard, collards, green beans, or spinach. Dried beans must be fully cooked. We like the crunch of the crisp-tender vegetables cooked only as long as it takes to cook the fritter, but if you would prefer them soft, parboil and thoroughly drain them before adding to the batter.

BASIC STIR-FRIED VEGETABLES

MAKES 4 SERVINGS

Stir-fried vegetables can be cooked in a large skillet or a wok. The advantage of cooking in a wok is that the vegetables can be pushed up the side of the wok and can receive less heat once they are almost tender. The advantage of stir-frying is that you can cook dinner in one utensil in a very short time. Although it is an Asian technique, it can be applied to dishes featuring other flavor traditions. Using a variety of colorful vegetables makes the dish more interesting, but the sauce determines its character. Here are some basic directions and three different sauces.

8 cups vegetables (see Note)
Sauce of your choice (recipes follow)
2 tablespoons vegetable oil
1 small onion or 4 green onions, chopped

2 garlic cloves, finely chopped
Salt and freshly milled black pepper
2 to 4 cups hot cooked rice, pasta, or other grain

Prepare the vegetables and have them ready to add. Prepare the sauce. Heat the oil in a large skillet or a wok. Add the onion and garlic and cook just until the aroma rises from the pan. Add the prepared vegetables and cook, stirring constantly, until they are crisp-tender, 5 to 7 minutes. Push the vegetables to the side of the pan. Add the sauce and cook, stirring constantly, until it is thickened, gradually combining the vegetables and the sauce. Taste and add salt and pepper, if necessary. Serve immediately with the rice.

NOTE: Thinly slice large vegetables into small pieces. Asparagus, broccoli, broccoli rabe, carrots, cauliflower, cooking greens, fresh peas, green beans, and winter squash should be parboiled and thoroughly drained before stir-frying. Bell peppers, green onions, mushrooms, snow and sugar snap peas, summer squash, tender greens, and zucchini can be sliced and cooked raw.

ASIAN SAUCE: Combine ¾ cup stock (see page 27); 1 tablespoon soy sauce; 1 tablespoon chopped peeled fresh ginger, or 1 teaspoon ground ginger; 2 teaspoons corn starch; 2 teaspoons toasted sesame oil; 1 teaspoon rice wine vinegar or white wine vinegar; and ¼ teaspoon hot red pepper flakes in a jar. Close tightly and shake until thoroughly mixed. Shake again before using.

MEDITERRANEAN SAUCE: Combine 1 cup finely chopped ripe plum tomatoes; ⅔ cup dry white wine; ¼ cup grated Parmesan cheese; 1 tablespoon chopped fresh basil, or 1 teaspoon dried; 1½ teaspoons fresh oregano, or ½ teaspoon dried; and 1 tablespoon all-purpose flour in a bowl. Stir until thoroughly mixed. Stir again before using.

SOUTHWESTERN SAUCE: Combine 1 cup stock (see page 27), 2 tablespoons cornmeal, 1 tablespoon chopped fresh cilantro, 2 to 4 teaspoons chili powder, and 1 teaspoon ground cumin in a jar. Close tightly and shake until thoroughly mixed. Shake again before using.

BASIC PILAF

MAKES 6 SERVINGS

This makes about six ¾-cup side servings. If you are serving it as a main dish, you should probably consider it four servings.

1½ cups white rice (see Note)
½ teaspoon salt
2 cups shredded carrots, zucchini, summer or winter squash, broccoli stalks, or asparagus or thinly sliced Swiss chard with stems, or a mixture

1 tablespoon olive oil
½ cup sliced green onions

Bring 3 cups water, the rice, and the salt to a boil in a 2-quart saucepan over high heat. Cover, reduce the heat to low, and cook for 15 minutes, or until the rice is just tender and all the water has been absorbed. Add the vegetables 5 minutes before the rice has finished cooking.

Heat the oil in a small skillet; add the onions and sauté until tender and lightly browned. When the rice has cooked, stir in the onions. Taste, add more salt, if necessary, and serve.

NOTE: If you would like to use one of the exciting new rice mixtures now on the market, just follow the package directions for 1½ cups of the rice and add the vegetables 5 minutes before the rice is fully cooked.

BASIC PASTA

Pasta and fresh vegetables are perfect partners. There are so many different combinations that can be created, we decided to just put the simplest recipe here and include others in the chapters that follow. Although the package will probably tell you that a pound of pasta makes eight servings, if you are serving it as a main course, you should probably figure on four. It rarely goes to waste.

4 cups vegetables (see Note)
1 pound pasta

2 to 3 cups hot tomato sauce
  (see pages 30–31)
Grated Parmigiano-Reggiano cheese

Prepare the vegetables and have them ready to add. Meanwhile, bring 3 to 4 quarts salted water to a boil in a large sauce pot over high heat.

Add the pasta and cook according to the package directions for al dente. Add less-tender vegetables (such as carrots, cauliflower, fresh peas, frozen artichoke hearts, and winter squash) with the pasta, moderately tender vegetables (such as chard, escarole, and green beans) about 3 to 4 minutes after the pasta, and quick-cooking vegetables (such as asparagus; bell peppers; broccoli; frozen green, snow, and sugar snap peas; and spinach) for the last 3 minutes. Drain thoroughly and serve with the tomato sauce and Parmigiano-Reggiano cheese.

NOTE: Asparagus, bell peppers, broccoli, cauliflower, and green beans should be cut into bite-sized pieces; carrots, cooking greens, summer and winter squash, and zucchini should be thinly sliced; and green, snow, and sugar snap peas can go in as they are.

There is almost no limit to what can go on top of a pizza—fresh or parboiled vegetables; meat, fish, or poultry; and any kind of cheese you crave.

BASIC PIZZA

MAKES 6 SERVINGS

2½ cups all-purpose flour
1 package quick-rising dry yeast
1 tablespoon sugar
¾ teaspoon salt
¾ cup very warm water
    (120° to 130°F)
1 tablespoon olive oil

2 cups vegetables (see Note), or a
    mixture of vegetables and fully
    cooked meat, poultry, or seafood
1 cup tomato sauce (see pages
    30–31)
1½ cups shredded mozzarella,
    Monterey Jack, Muenster, Cheddar,
    Fontina, or provolone or crumbled
    goat cheese, or a mixture

Combine 2 cups of the flour, the yeast, the sugar, and the salt in a large bowl. Add the water and oil; stir until a soft dough forms. Turn the dough onto a board; knead until smooth, adding any of the remaining ½ cup flour as needed. Oil the bowl; return the dough and let rise for 45 to 60 minutes, until doubled in volume.

Meanwhile, prepare the vegetables.

Shape the dough on a lightly oiled 12- to 14-inch pizza pan. Set aside for 15 minutes. Place an oven rack at the lowest position. Preheat the oven to 450°F.

Top the dough with the tomato sauce, vegetables, and cheese; bake for 15 to 20 minutes, until the crust has browned and the cheese is bubbly. Serve immediately.

NOTE: Cut large vegetables into small pieces. Asparagus, bell peppers, broccoli, broccoli rabe, carrots, cauliflower, cooking greens, fresh peas, green beans, summer and winter squash, and zucchini should be parboiled until crisp-tender. Onions and mushrooms are best if sautéed. All should be well drained.

BASIC STEW

MAKES 6 SERVINGS

Fresh vegetable stews make a hearty supper with little fuss. They can go from market basket to table in under a half hour. And, if you'd like to add a little more protein, you can serve the stew in a soup plate with a grilled chicken breast or fish fillet on top.

2 tablespoons olive oil or unsalted
    butter
2 large onions, chopped
2 to 4 garlic cloves, sliced
4 medium potatoes, peeled and cut
    into 1-inch pieces
4 medium carrots or turnips,
    cut into 1-inch pieces

1/4 cup all-purpose flour
3 cups quick-cooking vegetables such
    as broccoli, green beans, summer
    squash, spinach, zucchini, sugar snap
    peas, or precooked fresh or dried
    beans (see Note)
Chopped fresh herbs (optional)
Salt and freshly milled black pepper

Heat the oil in a large, heavy Dutch oven over medium heat. Add the onions and garlic and cook, stirring constantly, until lightly browned, about 4 minutes. Add the potatoes and carrots along with enough water to cover them by 1 inch. Cover the pot and bring the mixture to a boil over high heat. Reduce the heat to medium and cook for 12 to 15 minutes, until the vegetables are almost tender.

Stir 1/2 cup water into the flour; stir into the stew and cook until the stew is thickened. Add the quick-cooking vegetables, the fresh herbs, if using, and salt and pepper to taste. Cover and cook for 5 minutes, or just until the vegetables are crisp-tender.

NOTE: Cut large vegetables into small pieces.

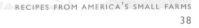

CHAPTER THREE

LUSCIOUS LEAVES

Tender or tough, pale and mild, or vibrant and pungent, all leaves are a plant's device for capturing the sunshine that it needs to begin photosynthesis. Fortunately for us, this crucial function doesn't interfere with a great many leaves being edible, tasty, nutritious, crunchy, and highly decorative.

Lettuce dates back to the third millennium B.C.E. Spinach is a comparative Johnny-come-lately on Western plates. Most sources show that it was brought to the West around the time of the Crusades, though it was used in Asia much earlier. Columbus brought the seeds of many kinds of greens to the New World, where they flourished in colonial kitchen gardens. Collards, which are native to many parts of the world, may have been brought to the New World by slaves.

Until the turn of the twentieth century, about one-third of the lettuce grown and sold in the United States was dark green or red. Fashion changed in the 1920s when iceberg lettuce was developed. At the same time, the development of the railroad made it possible for vegetables to be shipped long distances, and the sturdy iceberg was the only lettuce able to tolerate the journey. In the 1970s, lettuce, along with every other food, underwent scrutiny as tastes changed. Red-tinged European lettuces were introduced and exotic greens like arugula, corn salad, and Belgian endive began to appear in our markets. Kale, sorrel, and Swiss chard, once considered dull, became valued ingredients in the new American cuisine. In 1985, 'Red Sails,' the first all-red lettuce, was introduced. A few years later, 'Bright Lights' Swiss chard arrived on the scene with stems of vivid orange, glowing yellow, and shocking pink. Every year, new greens and rediscovered old ones appear in seed catalogs and on our plates.

Farmers, gardeners, and cooks have discovered edible leaves in many families in the botanical world. Once a plant is discovered to have tasty leaves, the plant breeders get to work. Four basic categories of lettuce have been developed: leaf lettuces that never form heads, creamy butterheads, crispheads like iceberg, and romaines. We can choose from thousands of lettuces, in a dazzling array of colors, shapes, sizes, and flavors. 'Forellenschluss,' an Austrian heirloom (its name means "trout's end"), is dark green speckled with burgundy; 'Red Fire' is as bright as its name suggests; 'Tom Thumb' forms a head that is small enough for a single serving. 'Lollo Rosa' and frisée are frillier lettuces, enjoyed for both their decorative qualities and the texture they add to salads. Chicory, improved over the centuries, yields an array of endives and radicchios whose slight bitterness has been mellowed. Sometimes, the older varieties of a plant deserve to be rediscovered. In most recipes, greens are interchangeable; see Mix and Match on page 60.

Most leafy greens are cool-season crops. Hot summer days cause the plants to produce seeds (which is known as bolting) and become bitter; lettuce and spinach are particularly susceptible. A notable exception is Swiss chard, which can withstand heat and humidity. The young leaves are great in salads, though they become tough as they age. Some other varieties, such as 'New Zealand' and 'Malabar' spinach, are heat lovers, but (to put it diplomatically) their taste is not universally loved. This all means that our salad bowls are often empty in the middle of summer, when we crave salads most. But farmers and breeders are working on heat-tolerant varieties ('Sierra' lettuce is one of the best) and growing methods, like shade covers and innovative irrigation systems, that help greens make it through summer.

As evenings get cool, our farmers have fewer fragile greens, but our CSA baskets are filled with kale and collards, which have the added advantage of tolerating frost. In fact, their taste is improved after they've gone through a few days of bitter cold. Leafy greens fall into two overlapping categories: those that are eaten raw and those that need to be cooked. Lettuce, arugula, chicories, and cresses are usually the stuff of salads, though wilted lettuce is occasionally seen and you'll find a few lettuce recipes in this chapter for those weeks when there's just too much for salad. Heavier greens, such as kale, collards, chard, and the mustards, can be eaten raw when they are very young and tender but benefit from cooking as they mature. The pungent flavor of kale and the sharpness of mustard greens are softened by cooking. Spinach does double duty; until it is very mature and tough, it's a perfect salad ingredient, but it also cooks up beautifully.

It's pretty easy to select great greens. They are perky and moist-looking, with no sign of dryness, discoloration, or damage. The major problem that occurs with leafy vegetables in the market is that their leaves become frayed and dried on the edges. Remember that anything that must be trimmed from greens or a head of lettuce is a loss, so select carefully.

It is important to prepare your greens for storage as soon as you get home from the CSA site or market. Even though you have selected the greens with the largest, freshest-looking leaves and checked to make sure the inner leaves are intact, they may look a little weary from travel. The crispness in greens is caused by moisture that's retained in the cells. Sometimes, this water evaporates during transit. Soaking the greens in cold water for a few minutes will often bring them back to life. However, if they still look perky, you don't have to wash your leafy greens before you put them away. Just make sure they're dry, remove any dead leaves, and store them in open plastic bags in the crisper of your refrigerator. If you have washed them, be sure to drain them well, as moisture will cause them to spoil quickly. Wrap the drained leaves in paper towels or put them in a reusable fabric crisping bag, and store them in the refrigerator. The fabric bags are available in housewares shops and can easily be made at home (see To Make a Crisping Bag, page 44).

Preparing greens for salads is easy. Tear the leaves; don't cut them with a knife, since the cut edges will quickly turn brown. Rinse your greens gently but thoroughly—no one likes sand in a salad—and dry them completely. The easiest way to dry salad greens is to leave them in a colander covered by a towel for a few hours, but that's no help when you need a salad in fifteen minutes. A salad spinner does the job quickly and efficiently, but if you don't have one, just shake the leaves in the colander, then lay them out in a single layer on paper towels and press another paper towel on top. This will take off most of the moisture, but you might still want to dry each leaf before adding it to the salad bowl (some people think that's overly fanatic—a little moisture on the lettuce leaves won't kill the salad).

Preparing Cooked

To prepare greens for cooking, rinse and drain, remove any tough stems and ribs, and cut the leaves into pieces or ribbons. The stems, particularly Swiss chard stems, can be used (in some parts of the world, the stems are used and the leaves discarded), but they need to be cooked for a few minutes more than the leaves. There are many ways to cook greens; the key is not to cook them too long. Here are some of the basics:

BRAISING is a quick way to "boil" your greens without overcooking them. Wilt the chopped greens in a large skillet with a little butter or oil. Add water or seasoned stock just to cover, and cook, covered, over low heat for 3 to 4 minutes, until the greens are tender but still slightly crisp. The more flavorful the stock, the more flavorful the greens will be.

SAUTÉING OR STIR-FRYING will tenderize and add flavor at the same time. Heat 1 tablespoon olive oil in a heavy skillet. Add 1 or 2 finely chopped garlic cloves and sauté for a minute or two. Add about 1 pound of chopped greens and toss quickly until the leaves are coated with oil. Cook, stirring constantly, until the greens are tender, 3 to 5 minutes. Season and serve.

MICROWAVING lets you cook greens in their serving dish without added fat or liquid. Place about 1 pound of washed but not dried chopped leaves in a 3-quart microwaveproof dish. Cover tightly; cook on high for 2 minutes, stir, and cook on high for another 2 to 3 minutes, until the greens are tender. Let stand for a few minutes, then season. When blessed with an abundance of greens, put some away for the winter.

WILTING is the method that retains the most nutrients. Rinse the greens, but don't dry them. Place them in a skillet with the moisture that is still clinging to the leaves. Add a pinch of salt for each pound of greens and cook, tossing gently, over medium heat for 2 to 3 minutes. Cover and cook for another 2 to 3 minutes, until they are tender and deeper in color. Very tough or mature greens may require another minute or two longer.

Preserving Greens

Freezing is easy and preserves the fresh flavor of greens. Most cooking greens freeze beautifully. Prepare them as for cooking (remove the tough ends and ribs) and chop roughly. Blanch in boiling water for 2 to 3 minutes (see page 00), drain thoroughly, and pack in plastic bags or freezer containers. You can't freeze lettuce because of its high moisture content; don't even try. But do try our Hot Lettuce Soup (page 46) and Lettuce Sandwich Spread (page 61) to reduce the bounty of lettuce in your refrigerator.

Greens Are Good for You

The darker the green, the more nutritious the leaves. Kale, chard, beet and turnip greens, arugula, and other members of the brassica and chenopodium family contain high levels of vitamins A, C, and K, calcium, and potassium, plus phytochemicals that are thought to fight cancer. These cancer-fighting antioxidants are also present in lettuces, which are high in vitamin A and potassium. Purslane, a sometimes cultivated weed with thick, sour-lemon-flavored leaves, has recently been shown to contain significant amounts of vitamin E and omega-3 fatty acids, both of which help fight heart disease. Many greens also provide folic acid, magnesium, and phosphorus. All greens are low in calories and fat, unless these are added in the cooking process.

To Make a Crisping Bag

Fabric crisping bags absorb the moisture from freshly rinsed greens, protect the greens from drying out in the refrigerator, and make convenient, reusable containers for storing your greens. To make one, purchase ½ yard of 36-inch-wide unbleached muslin or other coarsely woven fabric. Make sure it is 100 percent cotton. Wash and iron the fabric. Fold the fabric in half to make an 18-inch square with the right side of the fabric outside. Sew a ⅜-inch seam along each cut edge to make a bag. Trim off any fringes. Turn the bag inside out, press the seams, and make another seam down each side enclosing the rough edges of the fabric. Turn the bag right side out. Turn down the selvage edge to make a 1½-inch hem at the open top of the bag. Starting ¼ inch up from the selvage edge, secure the end and stitch around the open end of the bag to within 1 inch of the beginning of the seam. Secure the end of the stitching. Attach a 1½-yard piece of cording to a large safety pin and insert in the opening in the hem. Work the cording through the hem and out the opening where it went in. Remove the pin, knot the two ends of the cording—and your crisping bag is done.

BRUSCHETTA WITH BRAISED GREENS

MAKES 12 BRUSCHETTA

Bruschetta and crostini are wonderful hors d'oeuvres; the terms are used interchangeably outside Italy, though crostini are usually thinner slices of bread. You'll be surprised how many people—children included—are willing to eat their greens when they are served this way.

8 tablespoons olive oil
8 garlic cloves
1 pound mixed greens (such as kale, spinach, Swiss chard, and turnip, beet, or collard greens), rinsed, drained, and coarsely chopped
3½ cups chicken or vegetable stock

½ cup dry red wine (optional)
¼ teaspoon hot red pepper flakes
Salt
1 loaf of French or Italian bread, cut into 12 (¼-inch) slices
3 tablespoons grated Parmigiano-Reggiano

Heat 4 tablespoons of the oil in a large skillet over medium heat. Finely chop 2 of the garlic cloves and sauté until they begin to color. Add the chopped greens and sauté until they begin to soften, 2 to 3 minutes. (You may have to add the leaves in two batches if your skillet is not large enough, but the leaves will quickly decrease in volume.)

Add the stock and bring to a boil, then reduce the heat and cook, stirring occasionally, for about 20 minutes, or until most of the liquid is absorbed. If you're using the wine, add it during the last 5 minutes of the cooking time and keep stirring until most of the liquid is absorbed or evaporated. Add the red pepper flakes and salt to taste.

Meanwhile, toast the bread on both sides, brush with the remaining 4 tablespoons of oil. While the bread is toasting, cut the remaining 6 garlic cloves in half, then rub each slice with a half clove while it's still hot. When the greens are ready, transfer them to a sieve and let them drain for a minute or two. Place about 3 tablespoons of the braised greens on each slice of bread. Top with the Parmigiano-Reggiano cheese, and serve immediately or broil for a minute or two to melt the cheese before serving.

Salad Dos

(But Not All at Once)

- Mix flavors and textures: Mix a spicy arugula or bitter radicchio with bland and buttery varieties. Frilly frisées or Lollo Rosas work well with smooth spinach and oakleaf lettuce. And don't forget to blend your color palette—vivid reds are stunning against a background of pale green varieties.
- Add some crunch: Some greens, like Belgian endive, can serve the purpose; but think about toasted nuts, herb-flavored croutons, matchstick-sized carrots, shredded red or green cabbage, or sliced jicama.
- It doesn't all have to be raw: Sautéed mushrooms, roasted peppers, fried oysters, grilled chicken, or leeks dress up a salad.
- Boost the protein: Leafy greens contain incomplete protein, but the addition of items such as chickpeas or kidney beans, or bits of lamb, beef, poultry, or seafood, will make them a quality meal.
- Cheese fits perfectly: At the very last minute, right before the dressing, add cubes of sharp Cheddar or Gorgonzola, slices or balls of soft mozzarella, or curls of Parmigiano-Reggiano.
- Something sharp or salty is always good: A little diced prosciutto, capers, or pickled Vidalia onion goes a long way. Toss in a surprise: shavings of beets; chunks of pineapple, pears, or oranges; slices of sweet potato; handfuls of dried cranberries; or sunflower or pumpkin seeds.

HOT LETTUCE SOUP

MAKES 4 SERVINGS

Lettuce soups were sent to us by several CSAs. It is an ideal way to use large quantities of lettuce in the height of the season. For variety, garnish this with some chopped seeded tomato and crumbled bacon and call it BLT Soup.

2 small heads Boston lettuce (about 12 ounces), rinsed and drained
2 tablespoons unsalted butter

1 medium onion, thinly sliced
4 cups chicken or vegetable stock
Salt and freshly milled black pepper

Thinly slice enough lettuce to make 1 cup (see Chiffonade, page 48); set aside. Coarsely chop the remaining lettuce.

Heat the butter in a large saucepan over medium heat; add the onion and sauté until it just begins to brown, about 4 minutes. Add the chopped lettuce

Salad Don'ts

- Don't store greens in a plastic bag or other tight container until they are perfectly dry. The moisture will make them spoil quickly. If you are serving the greens right away, a little moisture won't hurt. It will only dilute the salad dressing a bit.
- Don't add the dressing until just before you serve the salad.
- The stronger the salad ingredients, the simpler the dressing should be. If you're adding fried clams, forget the raspberry-mustard dressing.
- Leftovers are fine, but don't kill a great salad by adding something that's past its prime.

and the stock to the saucepan. Bring to a boil, reduce the heat, and cook for 10 minutes.

Puree the lettuce mixture, half at a time, in a food processor or blender until smooth, transferring the blended mixture to another saucepan. Add salt and pepper to taste. Bring the soup just to a boil. Divide among 4 bowls and sprinkle with the reserved shredded lettuce; serve immediately.

Chiffonade

Frances Walker at Eatwell Farm in Winters, California, gave us these directions for making a chiffonade, or "ribbons," from herbs, lettuces, or cooking greens: First place 4 or 5 leaves on top of one another with the stems aligned. Trim off and discard the stems or reserve for cooking. Roll the leaves tightly in either direction. With a very sharp knife or scissors, thinly slice the rolled leaves. If using basil or other fragile herbs, do it at the last moment to prevent darkening.

DANDELION SOUP

MAKES 6 SERVINGS

This traditional Russian soup comes from Marina Yasnovsky, of the Carnegie Hill/Yorkville CSA on Seventy-fourth Street in Manhattan. This is best when served hot, as the bitterness increases when it is cold.

6 cups chicken stock (if using canned broth, use low-sodium)

6 cups chopped dandelion greens, or a mix of dandelion and sorrel, or spinach (about 6 ounces)

1 garlic clove, finely chopped

Salt and freshly milled black pepper

3 hard-cooked large eggs, chopped

3 Kirby cucumbers (or the equivalent), peeled and chopped

1 large potato, peeled, cooked, and coarsely chopped (optional)

3 green onions, chopped

Sour cream or plain yogurt

Chopped fresh dill or parsley (optional)

Bring the stock to a boil in a large saucepan. Add the greens, garlic, and salt and pepper to taste. Reduce the heat and cook until the greens are tender.

Meanwhile, to serve hot, divide the chopped egg, cucumbers, potato, if using, and green onions among 6 warm soup bowls.

When the greens are cooked, divide the soup among the bowls and garnish with sour cream or yogurt, and dill or parsley, if using.

Or, cool the soup to room temperature; assemble and serve warm within about a half hour.

CSAs frequently have a bountiful harvest of cooking greens, and members share the news when they discover good ways to prepare them. Robyn Harrison and Tom Hayden of New Mexico's Rhubarb Ranch recommend this traditional recipe from *The Food of Portugal,* by Jean Anderson. They leave out the sausage for a vegetarian version. They suggest adding an extra teaspoon of salt and your favorite herbs and spices. A combination of cumin and coriander is a good choice.

GREEN SOUP (CALDO VERDE)

MAKES 6 TO 8 SERVINGS

1 large yellow onion, peeled and minced fine

1 large garlic clove, peeled and minced

4 tablespoons olive oil

6 large Maine or Eastern potatoes, peeled and sliced thin

6 ounces chouriço, chorizo, pepperoni, or other dry garlicky sausage, sliced thin

2½ teaspoons salt, more or less

¼ teaspoon freshly milled black pepper

1 pound collard, kale, or turnip greens, washed, trimmed of coarse stems and veins, rolled crosswise, then sliced filament-thin (see Chiffonade, above)

Sauté the onion and garlic in 3 tablespoons of the oil in a large, heavy saucepan for 2 to 3 minutes over moderate heat until they begin to color and turn glassy. Do not brown or they will turn bitter. Add the potatoes and sauté, stirring constantly, 2 to 3 minutes, until they begin to color also. Add 2 quarts cold water, cover, and boil gently over moderate heat 20 to 25 minutes, until the potatoes are mushy. Meanwhile, fry the sausage in a medium-sized heavy skillet over low heat for 10 to 12 minutes, until most of the fat has cooked out; drain well and reserve.

When the potatoes are soft, remove the pan from the stove and with a potato masher, mash the potatoes right in the pan in the soup mixture. Add the sausage, salt, and pepper, return to moderate heat, cover, and simmer for 5 minutes. Add the collards and simmer uncovered for 5 minutes, until tender and the color of jade. Mix in the remaining tablespoon of olive oil, and taste the soup for salt and pepper. Ladle into large soup plates and serve as a main course accompanied by chunks of Broa (a crusty, dark Portuguese bread).

LETTUCE-AND-ORANGE SALAD

MAKES 6 SERVINGS

Early in the season, this salad is delicious when made from baby heirloom lettuce. Later on, you can enjoy it with broken leaves of mature romaine, Boston, or Bibb. It comes to us from Sunflower Fields Family Farm, in Postville, Iowa. Solveig Hanson, an apprentice at the farm, says, "We pick lettuces early in the morning—between six-thirty and eight-thirty—because it's cool then. If it's real hot when they're picked or if they get hot after they're picked, their life is shortened." The juice lost in slicing oranges is often wasted; here it forms the basis of the salad dressing.

3 large oranges, peeled and white membrane removed
8 radishes, thinly sliced
2 green onions, thinly sliced
6 cups baby heirloom lettuce leaves or torn mature lettuce leaves (about 6 ounces)

½ cup crumbled goat cheese or feta cheese
¼ cup sunflower kernels or coarsely chopped walnuts, toasted
3 tablespoons olive oil
2 tablespoons balsamic vinegar
Salt and freshly milled black pepper

Quarter and slice the oranges over a medium bowl, allowing both the slices and the juice to fall into the bowl. Remove membrane, if desired. Stir the radishes and green onions into the orange pieces.

Arrange the lettuce on a large serving platter. Transfer the orange mixture to the lettuce using a slotted spoon; reserve the orange juice. Sprinkle the salad with the cheese and sunflower kernels.

Whisk together ½ cup of the orange juice from the bowl, the oil, and the vinegar. Add salt and pepper to taste. Drizzle over the salad and serve.

This recipe comes from Terra Brockman, who works with her brother Henry of Henry's Farm, Congerville, Illinois. Wild (also known as rustic) arugula is an Italian heirloom form that's rarely available in supermarkets, but it's worth your while to look for it. It has the same peppery taste as conventional arugula, but its flavor is richer and more complex and its deeply serrated leaves add texture to salads and sandwiches. You can use cultivated arugula in this salad if you can't find the wild. Terra recommends using Parmigiano-Reggiano cheese for the best flavor.

WILD ARUGULA SALAD WITH MUSHROOMS

MAKES 6 SERVINGS

8 ounces wild arugula (about 8 cups loosely packed), rinsed and drained
8 ounces white mushrooms, thinly sliced (see Note)
6 tablespoons extra-virgin olive oil

2 tablespoons balsamic vinegar
1/2 teaspoon Dijon mustard
Salt and freshly milled black pepper
1 (6-ounce) piece Parmigiano-Reggiano cheese, at room temperature

Coarsely chop the arugula, reserving the spicy yellow flowers for garnish. Combine the chopped arugula and sliced mushrooms in a large bowl.

Whisk together the oil, vinegar, and mustard. Add salt and pepper to taste. Drizzle the mixture over the salad and toss to coat well. Shave thin strips of the cheese with a cheese shaver or vegetable peeler. Reserve your best strips for garnish; throw the rest into the salad and toss lightly.

Divide the salad among 6 serving plates and garnish with the reserved strips of cheese and the arugula flowers. Serve at room temperature.

NOTE: You may substitute porcini or other specialty mushrooms for the white mushrooms, but sauté them until tender first and let cool to room temperature.

Only the Best

Wholesome, fresh vegetables don't need a lot of fancy, processed ingredients. A lot of the products you'll find on gourmet market shelves are used more to make an impression than to make a great meal. But certain items do make a difference, and you'll find that if you use just a little of the best, the whole dish will taste better:

Oil: Extra-virgin olive oil and canola oil carry flavor better and never add an "off" taste

Vinegar: Balsamic vinegar adds rich flavor whenever it is used. Try other vinegars for special tastes; remember that just a splash is all you need.

Cheese: There's a world of difference between genuine Parmigiano-Reggiano cheese and the stuff in supermarket containers. This is one product where it always pays to go for the name brand.

FARM SALAD WITH ESCAROLE, WATERCRESS, PEARS, HAZELNUTS, AND BLUE CHEESE

MAKES 6 TO 8 SERVINGS

Executive chef Christopher Blobaum of the Surf and Sand Resort in Laguna Beach, California, told us, "We are very fortunate to have many small and large farms near by. We make this recipe with local, seasonal, organic produce." The extra time required to make the Roasted Pear Vinaigrette is well spent.

⅓ cup blanched whole hazelnuts (or use hazelnuts with skins)
Roasted Pear Vinaigrette (recipe follows)
1 head escarole, rinsed, drained, and leaves torn

2 bunches watercress, rinsed, drained, and trimmed of tough stems
4 Bosc pears, cored and sliced
Sea salt and freshly milled black pepper
¾ cup crumbled blue cheese

Preheat the oven to 350°F. Spread the hazelnuts on a rimmed baking sheet and roast until they begin to turn golden, 8 to 10 minutes. Set aside to cool slightly.

Prepare the vinaigrette; measure ¾ cup into a large bowl. Refrigerate the remaining vinaigrette for another use. Add the escarole, watercress, pears, hazelnuts, and sea salt and pepper to taste to the vinaigrette in the bowl and toss to combine.

Divide the escarole mixture among 6 to 8 chilled serving plates and top with the crumbled blue cheese.

ROASTED PEAR VINAIGRETTE: Preheat the oven to 375°F. Peel, quarter, and core 3 Bosc pears. Arrange the pears in a roasting pan; sprinkle with 1½ teaspoons sugar, and salt and freshly milled black pepper to taste. Roast for about twenty minutes, or until tender. Remove the pears to a blender. Add ½ cup pear or cider vinegar and ¼ cup apple juice to the roasting pan and stir to loosen the drippings from the pan. Add the mixture to the pears in the blender along with 1½ teaspoons honey, and vanilla extract to taste; set aside until cool. Blend until the pears are smooth, then, with the blender running, gradually add 1 cup light olive oil and ½ cup hazelnut oil. Taste and adjust the seasonings. Makes about 3 cups.

What's Mesclun?

Mesclun originated centuries ago around Nice in the south of France. The word "mesclun" (pronounced "mes-cloon"—although we are always amused when a farmers'-market customer asks for a bag of that terrific "mescaline") derives from the Niçoise dialect word "*mesclumo,*" meaning "a mixture." The traditional mixture has a bitter, spicy edge and includes various kinds of wild and cultivated endive (chicory), lamb's lettuce, and dandelion. Arugula, groundsel, chervil, purslane, and leaf lettuces also take part in the mix. In typical Yankee fashion, however, Americans threw out the traditional mix and redefined mesclun as any mix of leafy greens. This open-admissions policy—and the packaging and cheapening of ingredients by produce giants—leaves some yearning for the French original. . . . You can make your own mesclun mix, fancy or plain, spicy or mild, by buying the ingredients separately. Or, you can put your salad bowl in the capable hands of a good farmers' market or CSA farmer, who each week of the year picks the mix of leafy greens that are perfectly in season. A typical farmers'-market mesclun in autumn may include the four types of lettuces (Bibb, romaine, oakleaf, and crisphead), arugula, endive, red and green salad mustard, fennel, escarole, baby spinach, and chard, and tender wild greens such as lamb's-quarter and purslane. Fancy mesclun mixes also contain edible flowers such as bachelor's buttons, calendulas, chive blossoms, marigolds, nasturtiums, and violets.

—from Terra Brockman, Henry's Farm, Congerville, Illinois

Dressing in Style

Blue Cheese: Combine ½ cup olive oil, ¼ cup vinegar, ⅓ cup crumbled blue cheese, 2 tablespoons chopped fresh mild-flavored herbs, ½ teaspoon Worcestershire sauce, ¼ teaspoon salt, ¼ teaspoon sugar, ⅛ teaspoon ground black pepper, and 1 to 2 drops hot red pepper sauce in a screw-top jar. Shake well and store in the refrigerator. Bring to room temperature to serve. Makes 1 cup.

Buttermilk: Combine 1 cup buttermilk, ¼ cup grated cucumber, 2 tablespoons finely chopped green onion, 1 tablespoon Dijon mustard, 1 tablespoon chopped fresh herbs, 2 teaspoons lemon juice, ¼ teaspoon salt, and ¼ teaspoon ground black pepper in a screw-top jar. Shake well and store in the refrigerator. Makes 1⅓ cups.

Cilantro-Lime: Whisk together ½ cup olive oil, ¼ cup white balsamic vinegar, 2 tablespoons water, 2 tablespoons chopped fresh cilantro, 2 tablespoons lime juice, ¼ teaspoon salt, and ¼ teaspoon sugar in a small bowl. Store in the refrigerator. Makes 1 cup.

Creamy: Combine ¼ cup vinegar, ¼ cup sugar, 2 tablespoons light cream, 2 teaspoons fresh chives or other herb, salt and freshly milled black pepper in a small bowl; whisk vigorously until the sugar dissolves. Store in the refrigerator. Makes ½ cup.

Hoisin: Combine ½ cup olive oil, ¼ cup hoisin sauce, ¼ cup rice wine vinegar, 1 tablespoon finely chopped peeled fresh ginger, 1 teaspoon grated orange peel, and ¼ teaspoon hot red pepper flakes in a screw-top jar. Shake well and store in the refrigerator. Bring to room temperature to serve. Makes 1 cup.

Honey-Sesame-Mustard: Whisk together ⅓ cup vegetable oil, 2 tablespoons cider vinegar or rice wine vinegar, 2 tablespoons honey, 2 tablespoons hot mustard, 2 tablespoons toasted sesame seeds, 1 teaspoon finely chopped garlic or garlic scape, and salt to taste in a small bowl. Store in the refrigerator. Makes ⅔ cup.

Hot Peanut: Whisk together ¼ cup peanut butter, 3 tablespoons water, 2 tablespoons cider vinegar, 1 tablespoon honey, 1 tablespoon soy sauce, 2 teaspoons sesame oil, and hot red pepper flakes to taste in a small bowl until smooth. Add salt to taste. Store in the refrigerator. Makes ⅔ cup.

Mango: Puree 1 medium mango, sliced (about 1 cup), with 1 tablespoon vegetable oil, 1 tablespoon red wine vinegar, some chopped garlic, and salt and pepper to taste in a food processor. Add herbs and spices to taste. Try this with apricots and peaches as well. Store in the refrigerator. Makes 1 cup.

Orange-Ginger: Combine 3 tablespoons rice wine vinegar, 2 tablespoons orange juice concentrate, 1 tablespoon diced peeled fresh ginger, 1 tablespoon sesame oil, 2 teaspoons soy sauce or to taste, 2 teaspoons finely chopped garlic or garlic scape, and hot red pepper flakes to taste in a blender. Blend for about 1 minute, then add ¾ cup vegetable oil in a steady stream, blending until the mixture has emulsified. Store in the refrigerator. Makes 1 cup.

Tahini: Whisk together ¼ cup tahini, ¼ cup water, 2 tablespoons chopped green onion, 2 tablespoons chopped fresh parsley, 2 teaspoons chopped garlic scape, ¼ teaspoon salt, and ¼ teaspoon freshly milled black pepper in a small bowl until combined. Whisk in 2 tablespoons cider vinegar or white wine vinegar and 1 tablespoon lemon juice until smooth. Sprinkle with paprika or cayenne pepper. Store in the refrigerator. Makes ¾ cup.

Tomato: Combine 1 cup tomato juice, ¼ cup lemon juice or cider vinegar, 2 tablespoons finely chopped fresh chives and/or garlic scape, 1 teaspoon chopped fresh parsley or other herb, ¼ teaspoon salt, and ⅛ teaspoon ground black pepper in a screw-top jar. Shake well and store in the refrigerator. Use within several days. Makes 1¼ cups.

Vinaigrette: Add 1 halved garlic clove to ⅓ cup vinegar (balsamic or wine). Let it stand for at least 1 but not more than 24 hours. Remove the garlic; add ⅔ cup olive oil and season to taste with salt, freshly milled black pepper, and Worcestershire sauce or herbs. Store in the refrigerator. Bring to room temperature to serve. Makes 1 cup.

SWISS CHARD STEM GRATIN

MAKES 4 SERVINGS

This unusual recipe from Mariquita Farms in Watsonville, California, reminded us to tell you about our "Save the Stems" campaign. Most green leafy vegetable stems are just as delicious as the leaves and can be included in any dish you are making. All you have to do is start them in the cooking water two to three minutes before you add the leaves and they will be tender when the leaves are ready. Mariquita Farms is run by Julia Wiley, who lists her duties as Chief Executive Officer, E-mail Elf, Logistical Ultra-Babe, and Minister of Motherhood; and Andy Griffin, who has twenty years' experience in organic farming. Andy is also a prolific writer and chronicles his farm experiences in a beautiful magazine called *Roots* (see Resources for how to order). You might want to double the recipe for more generous servings.

Swiss chard stems from 2 large
   bunches, cut into 2-inch pieces
   (about 3 cups)
3 shallots, sliced
2 garlic cloves, finely chopped
$1/4$ cup olive oil

Salt and freshly milled black pepper
$1/8$ teaspoon ground nutmeg
$2/3$ cup heavy cream
$1/3$ cup dried bread crumbs
$1/3$ cup grated Parmesan cheese

Preheat the oven to 375°F. Butter a small casserole. In a large skillet, sauté the Swiss chard stems, shallots, and garlic in the oil over medium-high heat for about 2 minutes. Add salt and pepper to taste and the nutmeg; cook until the vegetables are tender, about another 4 minutes.

Transfer the vegetables to the buttered casserole. Drizzle with the cream. Combine the bread crumbs and cheese and sprinkle over the top. Bake for about 15 minutes, or until the crumb mixture begins to brown. Serve immediately.

This recipe was given to us by naturalist, author, and Chefs Collaborative supporter "Wildman" Steve Brill from his latest book, *The Wild Vegetarian Cookbook*. Brill leads public wild food and ecology tours throughout the greater New York area every weekend, and works with school classes and children's groups during the week. He's the author of several books but is best known for having been arrested and handcuffed by undercover park rangers for eating a dandelion in Central Park.

He told us, "Like the curries of India, Columbo is a traditional blend of herbs. Originating in Sri Lanka and Senegal, it migrated to the French Antilles islands of Martinique and Guadeloupe. A Haitian friend described it to me, I applied it to wild dandelions in America, and I'm offering it to you. Simple!"

DANDELION COLUMBO

MAKES 6 SERVINGS

6 cups dandelion leaves (picked in early spring, long before they flower, or late fall, when new growth appears—the seasons when they're at their best) (about 6 ounces)
1 medium cauliflower, sliced
6 garlic cloves, chopped
2 small hot peppers, seeds and ribs removed, or 1/4 teaspoon ground red pepper, or to taste
2 tablespoons peanut oil

1 cup unsweetened coconut milk
1/2 cup silken tofu
1 1/2 tablespoons mellow (light-colored) miso
1/2 teaspoon rum extract, or 2 tablespoons rum or any wild wine or sherry (optional)
1 teaspoon ground coriander
1 teaspoon ground turmeric
1 teaspoon dry mustard

Sauté the dandelions, cauliflower, garlic, and hot peppers in the peanut oil for 10 minutes.

Meanwhile, puree the coconut milk, tofu, 1/4 cup water, miso, rum extract, if using, coriander, turmeric, and mustard in a blender.

Mix the puree into the sautéed ingredients, bring to a boil, reduce the heat to low, cover, and cook another 10 minutes, or until the cauliflower is tender.

Kids and Greens

Wouldn't it be nice if kids loved greens? Some CSA members report that these simple tricks turn tots into greens lovers.

Start early. Kate, who has been a member of several CSAs, placed dabs of creamed spinach on the trays of her babies' high chairs and let them taste; she sometimes added a bit of brown sugar to the mix.

Put greens in unexpected places. Annie, a member from Miami, suggests that burgers are a good hiding place—she places creamy greens between the roll and the meat. She also throws a few tablespoons of chopped greens into fruit smoothies that she makes in her blender for breakfast.

Most kids love making pizza (see recipe, page 37) and adding toppings. If you supply some greens during the process, they'll often be used for their decorative properties, then eaten with pride.

Involve your kids in the kitchen whenever possible. Look for recipes that involve tearing greens, mixing, and pouring—even toddlers can handle these tasks.

SPINACH MATZO BALLS

MAKES 4 SERVINGS

Here's a recipe that CSA member Shelly Katz Beiderman of Manhattan makes with her daughter, Maille.

4 large eggs
1/4 cup olive, macadamia, or grapeseed oil
1/2 to 1 teaspoon salt
1/2 to 1 teaspoon freshly milled black pepper
1 cup matzo meal, maybe a little more
1 large bunch spinach, rinsed, drained, and finely chopped

Mix the eggs, the oil, 2 tablespoons water, the salt, and pepper in a large bowl until blended. Add the matzo meal and stir until it is well mixed; the mixture should be gooey rather than dry, but if it is still powdery, add an additional tablespoon or two of water until all the matzo meal is incorporated. (If the spinach is not thoroughly drained, you will need to add less water.) Incorporate the spinach and mix thoroughly. Refrigerate for 2 to 4 hours.

Thirty to 50 minutes before serving, bring a big pot of water to a full boil. Using an ice cream scoop, two spoons, or your hands, form the matzo mixture into large balls and drop into the water. Cook for 30 to 50 minutes, depending on how big they are. The matzo balls freeze beautifully.

ORGANIC WARM GREENS WITH BALSAMIC VINAIGRETTE AND CHÈVRE

MAKES 4 SERVINGS

Chef Bev Shaffer, cooking school director of the Mustard Seed Market & Café in Akron and Solon, Ohio, contributed this recipe. She says, "This popular recipe from my Produce 101 classes is a delicious way to 'green up' organic Lacinato kale, which has a mild, tender flavor. This dish is a favorite with my culinary students."

¾ cup extra-virgin olive oil
½ cup balsamic vinegar
2 garlic cloves, pressed
2 teaspoons honey
½ teaspoon paprika
1½ cups sliced white or cremini mushrooms

3 cups Lacinato (Tuscan) kale, rinsed, drained, and torn into pieces (about 3 ounces)
2 cups mixed organic baby greens
Salt and freshly milled black pepper
8 to 12 ounces firm chèvre (goat cheese), thinly sliced or crumbled
¼ cup pistachios, toasted

Whisk together the oil, vinegar, garlic, honey, and paprika in a small bowl. Bring ¼ cup of the mixture to a boil in a medium saucepan over medium heat. Add the mushrooms and cook for 2 minutes. Add the kale and cook, stirring once or twice, just until it begins to wilt.

Toss the hot mixture with the baby greens in a large bowl; add salt and pepper to taste. Divide the greens among 4 serving plates; top with the chèvre and toasted pistachios. Serve immediately; whisk the remaining balsamic vinaigrette and pass to drizzle over the greens.

Mix and Match

Greens are versatile ingredients. If you don't have what the recipe calls for, there is almost always something else that can take its place. Here are some flavor categories to keep in mind when selecting an alternate green for salads or cooking. When including the sturdier cooking greens in salads, select only the baby leaves.

Mild and Sweet: Bibb, Boston, green-leaf, iceberg, mâche, oakleaf, red-leaf, and romaine lettuces

Mildly Flavorful: Beet greens, parsley, spinach, and Swiss chard

Spicy or Peppery: Arugula, collards, kale, mustard, turnip greens, dandelion greens, mizuna, and watercress

Slightly Bitter: Belgian endive, chicory, curly endive, escarole, frisée, radicchio, and tatsoi

Aromatic: Basil, cilantro, and mint

Unique: Purslane (lemony) and sorrel (sour)

MIXED GREENS, MIDEAST STYLE

MAKES 4 TO 6 SERVINGS

This versatile recipe was submitted by Sue Burnham of the Live Earth Farm CSA, Watsonville, California. She says, "This is a very forgiving recipe. I have used all dried herbs when fresh were not at hand. I have used more or less greens and tomatoes. I have used this recipe over rice, in calzone with pine nuts and feta cheese, and on top of pizza. It also freezes well."

8 ounces mixed cooking greens (about 8 cups loosely packed), rinsed and drained
2 tablespoons olive oil
1 large onion, chopped
8 to 10 garlic cloves, finely chopped
1/4 cup chopped fresh parsley
1/4 cup chopped fresh cilantro
2 tablespoons paprika
2 teaspoons ground cumin
1/8 to 1/4 teaspoon cayenne pepper (optional)
2 cups chopped canned tomatoes, with their juice
Salt

Lettuce Sandwich Spread

There are not many farmers' markets where we have bags of mesclun left over at the end of the day. But there was one Saturday when the rain was coming down so hard that all but the most devoted (or demented) customers stayed home. So I ended up taking home a dozen bags and soon realized I wasn't going to make a dent in them even if all I ate was salad. One evening, I just threw two bags of it into the food processor with a little oil and vinegar, spread the mixture on a slice of hearty wheat bread, and, voilà! An incredible sandwich and a way to use many bags of lettuce, watercress, or arugula. Here's how:

Rinse 8 ounces mesclun (about 8 cups loosely packed). Dry it thoroughly in a salad spinner or spread the leaves on a towel and gently roll it up. Put 1 to 2 garlic cloves and 1 hot Thai pepper, if desired, in the food processor and chop fine. Add the greens, 3 tablespoons olive oil, 1 tablespoon balsamic vinegar, and salt and freshly milled black pepper to taste. Pulse until the leaves are chopped but not liquefied. Spread the mixture thickly on a sandwich of your choice. It works well alone or with a slab of fresh mozzarella, sharp Cheddar, or Jarlsberg. For more flavor, add fresh herbs (cilantro is great) to the blender; or mix in capers or chopped olives before spreading on the sandwiches. Makes 6 sandwiches.

—from Terra Brockman, Henry's Farm, Congerville, Illinois

Coarsely chop the greens. Heat the oil in a large, heavy pot with a tight-fitting lid over medium heat. Sauté the onion and garlic for about 5 minutes, or until they are soft. Stir in the parsley, cilantro, paprika, cumin, and cayenne, if using; cook for 1 minute. Stir in the greens. (The greens will shrink as they wilt, so you can add them by the handful if they do not fit in the pot all at once.)

Turn the heat to high; stir in the tomatoes with their juice. Cover and bring to a boil, reduce the heat to medium, and let simmer, covered, stirring often to prevent sticking. After about 20 minutes, add salt to taste.

If the greens are tender, reduce the heat to low, and simmer, uncovered, stirring frequently, until very little liquid remains. Do not leave them unattended; they scorch easily.

SWISS CHARD WITH GOLDEN RAISINS AND PINE NUTS

MAKES 4 SERVINGS

Richard and Mary Anne Erickson, chefs and owners of Blue Mountain Bistro in Woodstock, New York, contributed this recipe. They told us, "Swiss chard is one of the most popular leafy greens in Mediterranean countries. It is sturdy, stands up well to the heat of cooking, and is delicious. Spinach, kale, or a mixture of leafy greens can also be used in place of Swiss chard in this recipe. This makes a great first course or side dish and could be served over grilled or fried bread as an appetizer."

2 pounds Swiss chard, rinsed and drained
1/4 cup olive oil
1/4 cup golden raisins, soaked in warm water

2 to 3 tablespoons chopped garlic
2 anchovies, finely chopped (optional)
2 tablespoons sherry vinegar (optional)
Salt and freshly milled black pepper
1/4 cup pine nuts, toasted

Remove the Swiss chard greens and chop the stems into small pieces; keep separate. Heat the oil in a large, straight-sided skillet. Add the stems and a few tablespoons of water; cover and cook for 3 to 4 minutes. Uncover and continue cooking until the moisture has evaporated.

Add the Swiss chard greens, raisins, garlic, anchovies, if using, vinegar, if using, and salt and pepper to taste. Cook, covered, until the greens are tender, 3 to 4 minutes. Garnish with the toasted pine nuts and serve.

Meet the Farmer

Henry's Farm, Congerville, Illinois

After many years living in other cultures (Israel, Japan, Nepal, and Japan again), Henry Brockman realized that what was important was a simple, honest living that respected the earth and contributed to the health and well-being of others, "be they humans or rabbits, earthworms or soil microbes, oak trees or algae."

By working the land, Henry is able to be in intimate daily contact with the soil and the seasons —and with his family. "I became a farmer," Henry states, "because it was the only thing that made sense. I feed my family and other families without hurting the environment, I grow delicious and healthy food for people, and my kids know that when it's hot, you sweat and when it rains, you get wet."

Henry made the decision to make organic farming his life's work while still in Japan. That's where he met his wife, Hiroko, where they were married, and where, in 1990, their first child was born. When they first came back to the United States, they lived for a year in New York State, where they apprenticed with John Gorzynski, who grows organic vegetables for Manhattan's flagship Green Market in Union Square.

Henry was uncertain as to where his farming future would be. Then one day, on a trip back to visit his family in Congerville, Henry had an epiphany. He stuck a shovel into the ground, just as he had been doing in New York, and turned over the soil. For a long moment, he stared at the rich, black, loamy earth. That was it. He knew that this was where he had to be; this was the land he would farm.

And that's what Henry has been doing since 1993, building the soil, planting hundreds of kinds of vegetables, (more than 450 varieties in 2002), and enriching the lives of every person who eats them.

CHAPTER FOUR

THE CABBAGE CLAN

Cabbages have been cultivated for so long that their origin is obscured in the mists of time. However, their preference for cool, moist climates leads many food historians to nominate the fog-shrouded shores of northern Europe as a likely birthplace and the "sea kale" or "sea cabbage" that still grows wild there as a possible ancestor. Cabbages appear in Greek and Roman mythology but not in ancient Hebrew writings, lending support to the theory that they are one of the few Old World vegetables that migrated south and east rather than in the other directions.

The cabbages, members of the genus *Brassica,* grow prolifically, store well, and can be prepared with minimal equipment and energy. In the past, this co-operative spirit has led them to be typecast as food for hard times—peasant food. Fortunately, today, the brassicas appear on the best of menus—starring in main dishes and paired with seafood and poultry as well as with the traditional beef, pork, game, and sausages. A change in cooking technique has a lot to do with their new popularity. Cooks have learned that boiling cabbage-clan members until the aroma reaches the attic leaves them gray and unappealing, and that most brassicas are delicious served raw or briefly cooked. Not only is quick cooking convenient, but it leaves cabbages sweet, flavorful, slightly crunchy, and still colorful. In recent years, broccoli has moved to the top of the list of America's favorite green vegetables, and new cabbage-clan members (see Old and New Heads, page 66) are taking over more of the produce section.

The cabbage clan is hardy and grows abundantly in most parts of the United States. Cool-weather crops by nature, bok choy, broccoli, broccoli rabe, brussels sprouts, cauliflower, kohlrabi, green cabbage, Napa (Chinese) cabbage, red cabbage, and other specialty brassicas appear until the weather gets warm and then again in the fall. In fact, some of them are so hardy (kale, collards, brussels sprouts) that they are actually improved when they have survived a frost. Because they store so well, there's always some cabbage around for our Fourth of July coleslaw. Seed companies have introduced more Asian varieties to this country within the past decade, and plant breeders have produced both edible and ornamental cabbages to expand the family. CSA shares usually start the season with Asian cabbages, perfect for stir-frying with the green onions and baby vegetables that also appear at that time. As the weather gets warmer, small tender cabbages arrive to make the perfect coleslaw for summer picnics. By fall, the cabbages are so generous that members have to bring an extra bag for them, and it is time to bring out Grandma's recipe box and make the comfort foods we crave as the evenings get cool. With new shorter cooking times, they can be on the table in no time.

In this chapter, we are using the brassicas that are heads, expanded stems, or flowers, because they require similar cooking techniques. You will find some leafy members of the genus in chapter 3 and some roots in chapter 9. All are members of the good-for-you Cruciferae, or mustard, family. Whether you are selecting headed varieties or those such as broccoli, cauliflower, and specialty brassicas, look for firm, compact, slightly lustrous, brightly colored vegetables with no brown or black spots or wilting. Headed varieties should be heavy for their size, although Savoy cabbage will be slightly less heavy than the smooth cabbages because its leaves are looser, to accommodate their curliness. As to the brassicas that are theoretically stems and flowers, a quick check for flowers is often a clue to age and quality. Here are some guidelines: Broccoli should be a deep green and have no yellow flowers. Broccoli rabe may have a few yellow flowers if they are fresh-looking. Chinese kale (*gai lan*) is fine with fresh-looking white flowers. Choy Sum is the one that should have small yellow flowers, which are an interesting addition to any dish in which you would use a brassica. Despite cauliflower's name, the clusters

Old and New Heads

Several unfamiliar forms of broccoli and cauliflower have appeared recently. One of them is actually quite old; others are new hybrids.

Purple cauliflowers are not new, though they were seen only in home gardens during the past century. In colonial times, purple and even red cauliflowers were grown as often as green. They have the same taste and nutritional value as white ones.

Sprouting broccoli, sometimes called Romanesco or Italian asparagus (though it's totally unrelated to asparagus), is distinctive both in looks (yellow-green heads made up of tight spirals) and in taste (some people compare it to cashews). It's been known for two thousand years in Europe and was the broccoli of choice in Italy until the past century.

Broccoflower, a hybrid of broccoli and cauliflower, was hybridized in 1989 in Holland. Its cool chartreuse color and mild taste make it a good choice for salads.

Broccolini, trademarked in 1993, is the latest addition to the broccoli world. Though many people think it's a relative of asparagus, it's actually a cross between broccoli and leafy Chinese kale (*gai lan*). Broccolini, also known as baby broccoli, has a milder taste than either of its parents, and its thin stalks cook quickly and evenly.

should never resemble individual flowers; the surface should look bumpy and tightly packed. Any sign of separation is a clue that the head is past its prime.

After You Pick Up or Buy

Brassicas love a cool, moist climate, so all should be stored, unwashed and loosely wrapped, in the coldest part of the refrigerator. They will keep well in a brown paper bag, but plastic bags will cause them to spoil faster. If plastic is all you have, be sure to poke holes in it so moisture won't collect. Most CSAs deliver their brussels sprouts still on the central stalk looking like a tree of small cabbages. For easier storing, you can gently break each brussels sprout from the stalk by pressing down on it; remove any yellow or brown leaves before refrigerating in a paper bag. For best quality, plan to use broccoli, brussels sprouts, and cauliflower shortly after you bring them home; headed cabbages will maintain their quality for up to a week or two. Under special storage conditions, the firm-headed cabbages can be kept well into the winter. All seem to lose sweetness and gain sulfurousness with storage.

Preparing Uncooked

The headed cabbages, broccoli, cauliflower, and even brussels sprouts are delicious served uncooked. Because of the small visitors that may be attracted to organic vegetables, soak broccoli, cauliflower, and brussels sprouts in salted lukewarm water (4 cups water to 1/4 cup salt) for about 30 minutes; then trim them or cut the brussels sprouts in half and crisp them in ice water before using raw as crudités or in salads.

To prepare the headed cabbages, remove any tough or discolored outer leaves, and rinse the outside of the head. Although cabbages are so compact that there is seldom anything to remove from the interior, it doesn't hurt to quarter the head and rinse between the leaves with running cold water. Drain well, then trim out any dense central core and thinly slice the leaves for salad or slaw. To keep salads bright green and crunchy, don't toss them in dressing until you are ready to serve, as the acid in the dressing discolors the green leaves and causes vegetables to lose moisture. On the other hand, if you are making a slaw that is improved by taking in the flavor of the dressing and losing a little crispness, you might want to combine the cabbage and dressing and refrigerate the slaw, covered, for several hours or overnight.

Preparing Cooked

Organic broccoli, cauliflower, and brussels sprouts should be soaked in salted lukewarm water as directed above before cooking. However, they do not need to be crisped; just rinse off the salt water before they go into the saucepan, steamer, or skillet. We can't say it too often: Don't overcook your cabbages! All brassicas are high in sulfur-containing compounds or mustard oils. When they are cooked, volatile compounds are produced that let everyone in the house know you are cooking a member of the cabbage family. When they are overcooked, everyone in the neighborhood knows (see That Cabbage Smell, page 70). And, not only that, the vegetable in question loses its color, texture, and sweetness. This collection of assertive vegetables is remarkably easy to cook. They don't require any special attention—just keep the cooking time short and with the exception of steaming, keep the lid off. Here are some of the methods you can choose (see pages 6 to 14 for directions):

BLANCHING is useful when you want to partially cook broccoli, cauliflower, or brussels sprouts before using them on a vegetable platter or in a salad. It is also frequently called for when they are to be used in a quiche, frittata, or stir-fry where they might not cook sufficiently in the time needed for the other ingredients.

BOILING is the method to use if you want to dissipate some of the flavor intensity. Use lots of water, make sure the water is at a full boil before adding the vegetables, and cook, uncovered, until crisp-tender, no more than 5 to 8 minutes. Lift the vegetables from the water with a slotted spoon and allow them to drain completely in a colander before transferring them to a serving dish and adding sauce or seasonings. If you are cooking cauliflower, you might want to add a little lemon juice to keep the cauliflower white. If cooking brussels sprouts, broccoli or cauliflower with thick stems, or a whole cabbage, cut an X in the stem end for more even cooking.

BRAISING is a good way to add other flavors to the cabbages you are cooking. Although braising is usually long, slow cooking in a little liquid, in this case it is short, fast cooking in a little liquid. Once the broth or flavored liquid has returned to a boil, do not cook it longer than 5 minutes.

MICROWAVING works for one or two servings of broccoli or cauliflower florets, brussels sprouts, or sliced or shredded cabbages. Place them in a bowl with 2 tablespoons water, cover, and cook on high power for 3 to 5 minutes.

SAUTÉING OR STIR-FRYING is an excellent way to include brassicas in mixed-vegetable and meat combinations. It is best to blanch the vegetable to set the color and then add it at the end of the cooking process so that it doesn't overcook.

STEAMING is useful in cooking brassicas because their exposure to the heat can be controlled and they are not supersaturated with moisture. Because they must be covered for steaming, they will cook very quickly. Make sure the water has come to a complete boil in the steamer before adding the vegetables and steam them just until they are crisp-tender, 3 to 5 minutes.

Preserving

All the brassicas may be frozen for up to one year if held at 0°F. It is important to select quality produce to freeze; vegetables that are past their prime will not keep as well. Broccoli, cauliflower, and brussels sprouts should be soaked in salted water (see Preparing Uncooked, page 67) for 30 minutes, rinsed, and blanched for 3 to 5 minutes. Cabbages don't need to be soaked but should be cut into wedges or shredded and blanched for 3 to 5 minutes. All should be rinsed in cold water to cool quickly, thoroughly drained, and then packed in freezer containers. Be sure to label and date the packages.

Brassica Nutrition

No matter how you eat them, the cabbage clan is a healthy choice. Raw brassicas are high in fiber, vitamins A, B, and C, calcium, and potassium, and low in sodium and calories. Even after brief cooking, they maintain all of these benefits except vitamins B and C. Although cabbage-family members should be avoided by people with hypothyroidism, as cruciferous vegetables they are all part of the vegetable family thought to be of value in reducing the risk of cancer. Within the past ten years, medical researchers have recommended increased consumption of these tasty vegetables. And, as Grandma always said, "It couldn't hurt." We hope the recipes that follow will encourage you to include more bok choy, broccoli, broccoli rabe, brussels sprouts, cauliflower, kohlrabi, green cabbage, Napa (Chinese) cabbage, red cabbage, and other brassicas on your menu.

HIROKO'S FUSION CHOY WITH TAHINI-SOY DIP

MAKES 4 SERVINGS

Henry Brockman's wife, Hiroko, of Henry's Farm in Congerville, Illinois, came up with this recipe. The family says that it is a hit with everyone, especially the young children, who love dipping the stems into the sauce. Komatsuna is a beautiful blue-green Japanese choy that is longer, leafier, and more slender than the Chinese choys. It has a slightly more assertive flavor than bok choy or mei qing choy but is not at all bitter or sharp.

*1 medium head komatsuna
   (or 2 to 3 heads smaller choys)*
¼ cup tahini

*1 to 3 tablespoons lemon juice or
   water*
1 to 2 teaspoons soy sauce

Coarsely chop the komatsuna, leaving the stem portions about 4 inches long so that they will be a nice size for dipping.

Put the stems into a steamer for 2 minutes, then add the leaves and steam for 3 to 4 minutes, until crisp-tender. Drain, pressing lightly to remove the excess water. Meanwhile, combine the tahini, lemon juice, and soy sauce in a bowl.

Serve either by pouring the sauce over the komatsuna and tossing or by letting each person dip pieces into the tahini–soy sauce.

The Capay Valley, about ninety miles northeast of San Francisco, is home to at least twenty small organic farms, including Winter Creek Gardens. Winter Creek is owned by cousins Celso and Francisco and their uncle Sergio, long-time workers on organic farms in the valley, who seized the opportunity to buy their own farm in 2000. All are committed to growing food organically and sustainably. Their recipe for broccoli soup can be served hot or chilled.

FRESH BROCCOLI SOUP

MAKES 6 SERVINGS

1 ½ pounds broccoli
2 tablespoons olive oil
1 medium to large onion, chopped
2 garlic cloves, chopped
3 cups boiling water
2 tablespoons lemon juice
½ teaspoon dried thyme

½ teaspoon salt
½ teaspoon freshly milled black
    pepper
2 cups chicken or vegetable stock
1 cup whole milk
½ teaspoon ground nutmeg
Chopped fresh chives

Cut the tops of the broccoli into florets; peel the stems and cut into ¼-inch slices. Heat the oil in a large, heavy saucepan over medium heat. Add the broccoli, onion, and garlic; sauté until the onion is slightly softened, about 3 minutes.

Add the water, lemon juice, thyme, salt, and pepper. Cover and cook until the broccoli is very tender, about 10 minutes.

Puree in a blender with the chicken stock. Return the puree to the saucepan, add the milk and nutmeg, and heat through but do not boil. Taste and adjust the seasoning, if necessary. Garnish with chopped chives.

BIG SOUP

Robin Timm of Safe Home Farm in Platteville, Wisconsin, says, "When the garden is bursting with vegetables, it is time for Big Soup. Any and all veggies and herbs may enhance the flavor of this soup. It never comes out exactly the same. So, get yourself a big pot and make some Big Soup!" This soup freezes well. We enjoy our summer bounty in the middle of January, as we peruse the seed catalogs for next year's Big Soup. If you freeze the soup, do not add pasta until you reheat it.

2 large onions, chopped
3 garlic cloves, finely chopped
2 tablespoons olive oil
1 large green bell pepper, chopped
1 hot pepper (optional)
¼ cup dry sherry
1 small head cabbage, chopped
2 medium carrots, sliced
1 pound fresh green beans
2 cups cooked kidney beans
¼ cup chopped fresh parsley
1 tablespoon chopped fresh oregano

1 tablespoon chopped fresh savory or thyme
1 tablespoon vegetarian Worcestershire sauce
1 tablespoon tamari
Salt and freshly milled black pepper
1 pound broccoli, coarsely chopped
1 pound Swiss chard, leaves and stems
1 pound tomatoes, chopped
1 large zucchini, chopped
1 cup sliced white mushrooms
1 cup chopped fresh basil
2 cups small cooked pasta shapes

Sauté the onions and garlic in the oil in a large stockpot until fragrant, about 3 minutes; add the bell pepper, hot pepper, if using, and sherry; cook for 3 minutes.

Add 4 cups water and the cabbage, carrots, green beans, kidney beans, parsley, oregano, savory, Worcestershire sauce, tamari, and salt and black pepper to taste. Bring to a boil over high heat, then reduce the heat to low and cook for about 15 minutes—just until the veggies are heated through.

Add the broccoli, Swiss chard, tomatoes, zucchini, mushrooms, and basil and cook 5 more minutes, until the Swiss chard is bright green. Add the pasta before serving and heat through.

The term "coleslaw" comes from the German "*koolsla,*" meaning "cabbage salad." Coleslaw arrived in America with the earliest settlers, first appeared in print here in 1794 as "cold slaw" (a name that was still found in cookbooks until the mid–twentieth century), and in 1796 appeared in Amelia Simmons's *American Cookery,* the first cookbook written by an American. Through the centuries, the basic recipe has always allowed flexibility for the creative cook.

Here are just a few coleslaw variations for you to try. For each, start with 3 cups thinly sliced cabbage in a large bowl.

SESAME COLESLAW: Add 1½ cups shredded carrots and 1 cup thinly sliced spinach. Whisk together ¼ cup rice wine vinegar, 2 tablespoons sugar, 1 tablespoon finely chopped peeled fresh ginger, 2 teaspoons toasted sesame oil, and 1 teaspoon soy sauce. Toss with the cabbage mixture; season with salt and freshly milled black pepper and chill.

CAROLINA COLESLAW: Add 1 small onion and 1 small green bell pepper, both thinly sliced. Heat ¼ cup white wine vinegar, 3 tablespoons sugar, 3 tablespoons vegetable oil, 1 teaspoon dry mustard, and ¼ teaspoon celery seeds in a nonreactive saucepan until the dressing comes to a boil. Let cool completely. Toss with the cabbage mixture; season with salt and freshly milled black pepper and chill.

SPICY COLESLAW WITH CUMIN-LIME DRESSING: Add 2 large carrots, coarsely shredded; 1 small red bell pepper, cut into matchstick-sized strips; 1 small red onion, thinly sliced; and ¼ cup chopped fresh cilantro. Whisk together ¼ cup lime juice; 2 tablespoons olive oil; ¼ teaspoon ground cumin; 1 garlic clove, minced; and ¼ teaspoon hot red pepper sauce. Toss with the cabbage mixture; season with salt and freshly milled black pepper and chill.

ORANGE COLESLAW: Whisk together 3 tablespoons low-fat vanilla yogurt, 2 tablespoons low-fat mayonnaise, 2 tablespoons white wine vinegar, and 2 teaspoons grated orange peel. Toss with the cabbage; season with salt and freshly milled black pepper and chill.

COLESLAW COLLECTION

SAVOY CABBAGE AND LEMON SLAW: Whisk together ¼ cup low-fat (2%) buttermilk, ¼ cup low-fat mayonnaise, ¼ cup chopped fresh basil, 2 tablespoons grated onion, 1 teaspoon lemon juice, 1 teaspoon grated lemon peel, and 1 teaspoon chopped fresh summer savory. Toss with the cabbage; season with salt and freshly milled black pepper and chill.

CABBAGE AND APPLE SLAW: Add 1 large Granny Smith apple, peeled and finely chopped, 2 tablespoons finely chopped onion, and 2 tablespoons finely chopped fresh parsley. Whisk together ¾ cup plain yogurt, ¼ cup sour cream, and 2 tablespoons honey. Toss with the cabbage mixture; season with salt and freshly milled black pepper and chill.

CAULIFLOWER CHEESE PIE

MAKES 8 SERVINGS

This recipe was contributed by Urban Roots, a fifteen-acre certified organic farm located in Burlington, Vermont, and farmed by Jonathan Rappe.

Potato Crust (recipe follows)
2 large eggs
¼ cup milk
¾ to 1 teaspoon salt
¼ teaspoon freshly milled black pepper
3 tablespoons unsalted butter
1 cup chopped onions
1 garlic clove, finely chopped

1 medium cauliflower, broken into small florets
2 tablespoons chopped fresh parsley
1½ teaspoons chopped fresh basil, or ½ teaspoon dried
¾ teaspoon chopped fresh thyme, or ¼ teaspoon dried
1¾ cups grated Cheddar cheese
Paprika

Preheat the oven to 400°F. Generously oil a 9-inch pie pan. Prepare and bake the potato crust. Reduce the oven temperature to 350°F when the crust is done.

Meanwhile, beat together the eggs, milk, ½ teaspoon of the salt, and the pepper in a small bowl; set aside.

Melt the butter in a large skillet over medium heat. Add the onions, garlic, and ¼ to ½ teaspoon of the remaining salt; cook, stirring frequently, until lightly browned, about 5 minutes. Add the cauliflower, parsley, basil, and thyme; cook, covered, for 10 minutes, stirring occasionally. Remove from the heat.

Over the baked potato crust, layer half of the Cheddar cheese, then the cauliflower mixture, then the remaining cheese. Pour the milk mixture over the top and lightly dust with paprika. Bake for 35 to 40 minutes, until set.

POTATO CRUST: Place 2 firmly packed cups grated raw potatoes in a colander set over a bowl; toss the potatoes with ½ teaspoon salt and set aside for 10 minutes. Squeeze out the excess water. Combine the drained potatoes; 1 large egg, beaten; and ¼ cup grated onion in a medium bowl. Pat the potato mixture into the oiled pie pan, building up the sides of the crust with lightly floured fingers. Bake for 35 to 40 minutes, until golden brown, brushing the crust with oil after the first 20 minutes to crisp it.

BROCCOLI FLAN

MAKES 4 MAIN-DISH SERVINGS OR 6 SIDE-DISH SERVINGS

Feel free to experiment with other vegetables; you can use summer squash, any kind of greens, even leeks. Barbara Berger of Carnegie Hill/Yorkville CSA, in Manhattan, who submitted this recipe, suggests, "For a one-dish meal, add fresh crab, shrimp, or cut-up poultry."

1 pound broccoli, coarsely chopped
½ medium onion, thinly sliced
4 large eggs
2 cups grated Swiss or Jarlsberg cheese
1½ teaspoons chopped fresh oregano, or ½ teaspoon dried
1½ teaspoons chopped fresh basil, or ½ teaspoon dried
½ teaspoon salt
¼ teaspoon freshly milled black pepper

Preheat the oven to 325°F. Lightly grease a 1½-quart baking dish. Steam the broccoli and onion until just tender. Do not overcook. Drain well.

Meanwhile, beat the eggs in a large bowl and fold in the cheese. Add the broccoli mixture to the eggs along with the oregano, basil, salt, and pepper.

Transfer the mixture to the greased baking dish and bake, covered, for 30 to 40 minutes, until set.

STRIPED BASS AND SCALLOPS WITH BRAISED CABBAGE AND GREMOLATA BUTTER

MAKES 4 SERVINGS

This recipe is from Peter Hoffman, who is the national chair of Chefs Collaborative and the chef and owner of Savoy Restaurant in New York City. He recommends using Taylor Bay scallops if you can get them.

Gremolata Butter (recipe follows)
2 tablespoons olive oil
3 cups 1-inch strips Savoy cabbage
1 cup ½-inch cubes Jerusalem
   artichokes or fingerling potatoes

¼ cup vegetable or fish stock
¼ cup dry white wine
12 to 16 ounces striped bass fillets
12 Taylor Bay scallops or littleneck
   clams

Preheat the oven to 375°F. Prepare the gremolata butter.

Heat 1 tablespoon of the oil in a large saucepan over medium heat. Add the cabbage and Jerusalem artichoke pieces and sauté briefly. Add the stock and wine; reduce the heat to low, cover, and simmer for 8 minutes.

Meanwhile, heat the remaining 1 tablespoon olive oil in an ovenproof skillet. Add the pieces of fish, skin side down; sauté until golden brown. Turn the fish and place the skillet in the oven for 5 minutes.

Add the scallops to the vegetables and cook for 2 minutes, or until the scallops open. Remove the scallops to a bowl. Add the gremolata butter to the broth in the saucepan; swirl to combine the broth and melted butter.

To serve, divide the vegetables and broth among 4 warm soup plates. Arrange the fish and scallops on top. Sprinkle with the reserved gremolata mixture and serve.

GREMOLATA BUTTER: Combine 2 tablespoons coarsely chopped fresh parsley, 2 teaspoons finely grated lemon peel, 1 teaspoon finely grated orange peel, and 1 small garlic clove, finely chopped, in a small bowl. Set aside 2 teaspoons of the mixture for garnish. Stir the remaining mixture into 4 tablespoons softened unsalted butter; add salt to taste and set aside.

Broccoli Salads

No one has coined a snappy name like coleslaw for cold broccoli salads, but that doesn't make them any less delicious. Here are a few to try. Slice 1½ pounds of broccoli and cook using any of the methods suggested on pages 6 to 14 until crisp-tender. Drain well and combine with any of the following (each salad serves 4):

Bacon and Onion: Cook 4 slices of bacon until crisp; crumble. Whisk together ⅔ cup olive oil and 3 tablespoons red wine vinegar until blended; add 1 cup chopped red onions. Season with salt and freshly milled black pepper. Toss with the broccoli and bacon until well coated. Garnish with sunflower seeds.

Sesame: Whisk together 2 tablespoons soy sauce, 2 tablespoons rice wine vinegar, 2 tablespoons Asian sesame oil, and 2 tablespoons honey in a large bowl. Toast ½ cup sesame seeds in a heavy skillet; let cool. Mix the broccoli and half of the sesame seeds into the dressing. Marinate at room temperature for 30 minutes to 2 hours, tossing occasionally. Transfer the broccoli to a platter, pour the dressing over, and sprinkle with the remaining sesame seeds.

Walnuts, Raisins, and Red Onion: Mix ½ cup mayonnaise or plain low-fat yogurt, ¼ cup sugar, and 1 tablespoon vinegar until blended; refrigerate overnight. Toss with the broccoli, ¼ cup chopped walnuts, ¼ cup raisins, and ¼ cup chopped red onion.

Pasta or Wild Rice: Mix 2 cups cooked pasta or wild rice with the broccoli; add ½ cup sautéed mushrooms. Dress with Vinaigrette (page 55) or with 2 tablespoons mayonnaise. Season with chopped fresh herbs, green onions, salt, and pepper. Add 2 tablespoons pine nuts, if desired.

Cherry Tomatoes, Nuts, and Cheese: Whisk together 2 teaspoons Dijon mustard, 3 tablespoons rice wine vinegar, 1 tablespoon olive oil, and 2 tablespoons chopped fresh herbs. Toss with the broccoli, 2 cups halved cherry tomatoes, ½ cup chopped nuts (walnuts, almonds, or pecans), and ½ cup crumbled cheese (blue cheese, goat cheese, or Cheddar). Toss to coat. Season with salt and freshly milled black pepper. Chill.

Chicken-Herb: Mix the broccoli with 3 cups chopped cooked chicken, ¼ cup chopped fresh parsley or dill, and ¼ cup sour cream. Add salt to taste.

A Narrow Bridge

Narrow Bridge Farm is located on four scenic acres just five miles from downtown Ithaca, New York. It is run by Jon Thorne (he mostly goes by his Hebrew nickname, Yoni), who grew up in Southern California and has been farming since 1996, and Tali Adini, who grew up in Philadelphia and moved to Israel at age eighteen. In the early 1990s, they traveled to Southeast Asia and beyond for a year. It was in New Zealand that they became interested in organic farming. Upon returning to the United States, they worked and apprenticed in California, the Hudson Valley, and Ithaca for several years. The name of their farm is derived from a Talmudic adage, "All the world is a narrow bridge, and the most important thing is not to be afraid." Tali says it's a perfect description of the precariousness of farming—the balance that farmers must strike between their carefully planned work and the effects of the elements. What makes the name even more appropriate is that the word for "most important thing" in Hebrew, *ikar,* is a homonym for the word "farmer"!

BAKED BRUSSELS SPROUTS IN WHITE SAUCE

MAKES 4 SERVINGS

Edith Harnik, a founding member of the Carnegie Hill/Yorkville CSA, firmly believes in the adage "Reduce, reuse, recycle"; she even washes and reuses Saran wrap. She couldn't bear to throw away the tall stalks that bore our fresh brussels sprouts. So she trimmed off the toughest part—up to the point that she could cut with a sharp knife—and sliced the rest into chunks. She boiled these slices of brussels sprouts stalk until they were tender, then sliced them open—and sure enough, she found a soft pulp inside that was quite delicious. In the following recipe, she sometimes substitutes *Einbrenn* (see page 79) for the white sauce.

1 pound brussels sprouts, trimmed,
   brown leaves removed
3 tablespoons unsalted butter
3 tablespoons all-purpose flour

½ cup milk, heated until almost scalded
Salt and freshly milled black pepper
¼ cup fresh bread crumbs, lightly
   toasted

Cut an "X" into the base of each brussels sprout. Steam or boil them until crisp-tender, then drain and put into a small baking dish.

Preheat oven to 350°F. Melt the butter in a small saucepan; whisk in the flour and stir until combined, then cook for a minute or two. Pour in the hot milk and continue whisking until the mixture is fully blended and begins to thicken. Add salt and epper to taste. Pour the white sauce over the brussels sprouts, then top with the bread crumbs.

Bake about 15 minutes, until bubbly and the top is browned.

In German cooking, a light sauce called *Einbrenn* is often used for simple vegetable dishes. The vegetable cooking liquid, rather than milk or cream, is used as the base of the sauce, which conserves both flavor and vitamins that would otherwise be lost. This is Leslie Ackerman's interpretation of her mother's (Grandma Betty's) *Kohlrabi mit Einbrenn*. Leslie is a member of Narrow Bridge Farm, Ithaca, New York.

KOHLRABI *EINBRENN*

MAKES 3 TO 4 SIDE-DISH SERVINGS

4 small kohlrabi with leaves
1½ cups stock or water
1 tablespoon vegetable oil or unsalted
    butter
1 tablespoon all-purpose flour

Salt and freshly milled black pepper
⅛ to ¼ teaspoon ground nutmeg or
    2 tablespoons chopped fresh savory
    (optional)

Peel the kohlrabi bulbs and cut into ¼-inch slices; reserve the leaves. Bring the stock to a boil in a medium saucepan, add the kohlrabi slices, and simmer, covered, for 10 to 15 minutes, until just tender. Remove the slices from the simmering liquid with a slotted spoon and set aside.

Add the kohlrabi leaves to the pot and simmer, covered, for 5 to 7 minutes, until tender. Drain the leaves, reserving 1 cup cooking liquid; keep the liquid hot. Chop the leaves.

Heat the oil in a saucepan, then whisk in the flour and cook the mixture for about 1 minute. Add the reserved hot cooking liquid, whisking to avoid lumps. Simmer, uncovered, for several minutes, until the sauce thickens slightly. Add the cooked kohlrabi slices and leaves and simmer for a minute or two. Season with salt and pepper and, if desired, nutmeg or savory.

Stuffed Cabbage

There are many ways to stuff a cabbage, but the basics are the same. Here's an easy, all-purpose stuffing and three ways to present it.

Stuffing: Sauté 8 ounces ground beef, lamb, or turkey, or mushrooms, chopped, and 1 small onion, chopped, in 1 teaspoon olive oil in a large skillet over medium heat until the meat is no longer pink. Stir in 1 cup water, ½ cup white rice, ½ teaspoon salt, and ½ teaspoon dried basil or dill. Cover and cook over low heat until the rice is tender and all the liquid is absorbed, about 15 minutes. See the other stuffing recipes on page 164.

Stuffed Cabbage 1: Remove 12 large leaves from a head of cabbage and boil them in a large pot of water for 5 minutes. Drain well and flatten the large veins with a spatula. Divide the stuffing among the leaves; with each leaf, fold the sides over the stuffing and roll up. Bring 2 cups tomato sauce (see Basic Tomato Sauces, page 30) to a boil in a large skillet. Place the stuffed cabbage rolls, seam side down, in the sauce; cover and simmer for 10 minutes.

Stuffed Cabbage 2: Preheat the oven to 400°F. Remove 12 large leaves from a head of cabbage and boil them in a large pot of water for 5 minutes. Drain well and line a buttered 1-quart casserole with 4 of the leaves. Add half of the stuffing, 4 more leaves, the remaining stuffing, and the remaining 4 leaves. Cover and bake until heated through, 20 to 25 minutes. Unmold onto a platter and cut into quarters, or serve from the casserole. Serve with 2 cups heated tomato sauce (see Basic Tomato Sauces, page 30).

Stuffed Cabbage 3: Preheat the oven to 400°F. Turn back 4 to 6 large outer leaves from a head of cabbage and carve out a hollow in the center of the head big enough to hold the stuffing. Invert the cabbage into a large pot of boiling water. Return the water to a boil and cook until the cabbage is crisp-tender, about 5 minutes. Drain well and stuff with the meat mixture. Turn the outer leaves back over the stuffing. Wrap the cabbage tightly in aluminum foil, place in a baking pan, and bake for 20 to 25 minutes, until heated through. Unwrap and place in a vegetable bowl. Cut in quarters and serve with 2 cups heated tomato sauce (see Basic Tomato Sauces, page 30).

Just assemble this traditional side dish and let it mind itself in the oven while you do other things. Joanne Hayes, member of the Carnegie Hill/Yorkville CSA in Manhattan and coeditor of this book, says, "The tender new organic red cabbage we get from our farm makes the best sweet-and-sour cabbage I have ever had. I sometimes just make a sandwich of sweet-and-sour red cabbage and cheese."

EASY SWEET-AND-SOUR RED CABBAGE

MAKES 6 SERVINGS

1 tablespoon unsalted butter
1 large onion, thinly sliced
1 ½ pounds red cabbage, thinly sliced
  (about 6 cups loosely packed)
1 large Golden Delicious apple, thinly
  sliced

⅓ cup cider vinegar
⅓ cup sugar
¾ teaspoon salt
¼ teaspoon freshly milled black
  pepper

Preheat the oven to 375°F. Melt the butter in a large Dutch oven over medium heat. Add the onion and sauté until golden, 3 to 5 minutes. Remove from the heat and stir in the cabbage and apple.

Whisk together the vinegar, sugar, salt, and pepper in a cup until the sugar is dissolved. Pour over the cabbage mixture. Cover and cook in the oven for about 45 minutes, or until the cabbage is crisp-tender. Stir thoroughly; taste and adjust the seasonings.

Broccoli Sauces

Cheese Sauce: Melt 2 tablespoons unsalted butter in a heavy pan. Add 2 tablespoons all-purpose flour and whisk for 2 to 3 minutes, until it is combined. Heat 1 cup milk until almost—but not quite—scalded. Add to the flour-butter mixture and whisk until completely smooth, about 8 minutes. Add ¼ cup finely grated Cheddar cheese; stir over low heat until the cheese melts. Season with salt, freshly milled black pepper, and ground nutmeg.

Horseradish Sauce: Mix 3 tablespoons sour cream with 2 tablespoons prepared horseradish; add 1 tablespoon chopped fresh chives. Toss with hot broccoli.

BROCCOLI RABE SAUTÉ

MAKES 6 SERVINGS

Related to broccoli, rabe has a slightly sharp flavor that can become bitter if overcooked. This traditional Italian preparation makes broccoli rabe shine. This recipe comes from Jerry Spencer of Mount Laurel Organic Gardens in Birmingham, Alabama.

1 large bunch broccoli rabe
2 tablespoons extra-virgin olive oil
2 garlic cloves, thinly sliced

1 ½ tablespoons lemon juice
Salt and freshly milled black pepper

Rinse the broccoli rabe carefully, removing and discarding the large stems. Drain well.

Heat the oil in a large saucepan over medium-low heat; add the garlic and sauté until golden brown, about 1 minute. Add the broccoli rabe; increase the heat to medium-high. Cover and cook, stirring frequently, until the rabe is wilted, about 5 minutes.

Season with the lemon juice, and salt and pepper to taste.

VARIATION: Sauté a sliced red bell pepper with the broccoli rabe and toss it with cooked penne pasta (8 ounces before cooking) and a splash of heavy cream for a satisfying main course.

The Joy of Eating

Jerry Spencer, who runs Mount Laurel Organic Gardens in Birmingham, Alabama, believes that Mount Laurel is about the joy of eating. "Any good chef will tell you that the first step in great cooking is to buy locally grown produce," he says. "This is because local is fresher" ("Our vegetables are harvested and in your home within about twenty-four hours," says Jerry) and because he selects varieties for taste alone, not for shipping ability or shelf life. Cooking classes, taught by a chef, are held regularly at the farm so that members can improve their cooking skills and learn how to use farm-fresh produce. The farm also operates a children's farm camp, where teachers bring students for a day at the farm. Special events such as a spring farm-opening salad fair, with more than fifty salad components; a tomato festival in August; and a fall harvest festival featuring cooking greens and pumpkins focus on the best that the farm has to offer.

CHAPTER FIVE

THE ONION FAMILY

The onion family demands attention! You would never guess these pungent edible bulbs of the genus *Allium* were really members of the amaryllis, or lily, family. Onions, garlic, leeks, and their cousins have been adding character to the world's cooking since the ancient Egyptians wrote about them and probably since prehistory. Native to Central and Southwest Asia, where they still grow wild, they traveled to the Mediterranean as part of the personal supplies of early traders and settled in wherever they were carried. Bulb onions, leeks, and garlic were brought to what is now Europe and Britain by the Roman army, and several centuries later, shallots were introduced to these areas by returning Crusaders.

Although in some areas eating the bulbs and greens was forbidden or discouraged by certain classes, who found a hint of onion or garlic on the breath offensive, alliums were embraced by working people the world over. Then, as now, they were eaten raw as well as in cooked foods, and medicinal and supernatural powers were attributed to them. The onion family is certainly one of the most important elements of the world's seasoning repertoire. There is no culture that doesn't use onions or garlic to flavor their menu. It is often said that the welcoming aroma of onions frying means you're home and dinner is almost ready.

In the Field

There are so many different members of the onion family that they are represented each week in our CSA. Whether we get red, yellow, white, green, sweet, boiling, or pearl onions, chives, cipolline, garlic, garlic scape, shallots, or leeks, we always have something to provide that incomparable flavor and aroma to our week's meals. One of our special celebrations is in honor of the garlic harvest. Members are invited to go to the farm and help, and there are so many volunteers that the job is done in no time. Although the garlic has to stay at the farm and dry for several weeks, we can each look forward to getting a handful of heads just in time to season our Thanksgiving turkey. Onions are considered either "fresh" or "keepers" (or "storage onions"). Just like our garlic, most red, white, and yellow onions (including cipolline) are dried for storage after harvest, whether they are large or small.

Selecting the Best

Onions that have been dried should be firm and fresh-smelling with crisp, dry skins. Avoid ones that are sprouting, sooty-looking, greenish, or slightly translucent in spots, or have woody stems; they are past their prime. Green onions and scallions should be crisp with bright green leaves, luminous white bulbs, and no sign of wilting or wetness. Leeks should have bright greens and white whites with no yellowing or wilting. They should be firm and straight, with no sign of limpness and no slime at the roots. Shallots should have dry papery skins with no sprouts or soft spots.

After You Pick Up or Buy

Storage onions, no matter their size, should be kept in a cool, dry place where there is plenty of air circulation. The refrigerator is not usually the best choice because of its moisture. Most of all, they should never be stored near potatoes, as the moisture from the potatoes will cause onions to sprout and to mold. In the ideal climate, properly dried storage onions can last several months. If onions start to sprout, try to use them quickly and remove and discard the green core caused by the sprouting because it is sometimes bitter.

At the beginning of the onion harvest season, we sometimes get fresh onions in our CSA shares before they have been dried, but that would be a rare commodity in markets. Sweet onions are usually sold fresh, as are green onions, scallions, leeks, ramps, garlic scape, green garlic, chives, and garlic chives. Fresh onions and their cousins are perishable; they should be placed in breathable plastic bags or ones with holes snipped in them, refrigerated, and used in three or four days.

Preparing Uncooked

To prepare raw onions, simply remove the papery outer layer and, if they have started to sprout, any green in the center. Unless you need perfect rounds, it is much easier to slice or chop onions if you halve them first. They are then ready to use in salads, on sandwiches, or as an ingredient in relishes and salsas. Alliums with greens should be trimmed at the point where the greens get tough or dried-looking. The rest may be used with the bulb. Because of their "bite" and pungent aroma, raw onions elicit strong feelings from most people—they either love them or hate them. Sweet onions are a seasonal option that is more likely to be a crowd pleaser.

Preparing Cooked

Because of the different chemical changes involved, alliums have a different flavor when raw, cooked by dry heat, or cooked by moist heat. Much of the aroma and flavor can be volatilized by cooking. To get rid of a lot of the flavor and aroma, use a lot of water and no lid; to retain the flavor, use little or no liquid and a lid. All alliums become sweeter and more mellow when cooked. Although you could steam or microwave onions, we don't recommend it except for scallions and green onions. There are so many more interesting things you can do with them.

BLANCHING is a quick trick for removing the skins from boiling and pearl onions and cipolline before boiling, glazing, or roasting.

BOILING is a traditional method for preparing small onions. As a matter of fact, walnut-sized onions are called boiling onions whether they are red, white, or yellow. Hazelnut-sized pearl onions are another good choice for boiling, as are the slightly larger, flat Italian onions called cipolline. All should be peeled and cooked over medium heat until crisp-tender in a covered pan with just enough boiling salted water to cover them. This should take 12 to 15 minutes for pearl onions and 20 to 25 for the larger ones. Watch to make sure there is always enough water, and drain them as soon as they are cooked. Boiled onions in cream sauce are an essential for New England holiday dinners.

BRAISING is a perfect way to cook onions when you have the oven on for a roast. Just put them in a heavy, ovenproof casserole with a little broth, wine, or fruit juice. Season them with salt and freshly milled black pepper to taste and cook them covered until they are crisp-tender. The timing will, of course, vary depending upon the size of the onions and the temperature you are using for the meat; check for doneness every 15 minutes.

DEEP-FRYING is a bit messy but produces some onion classics. Deep-fried onion rings, flowers, and loaves are bringing people back to restaurants all across the country. You might want to do it occasionally as a special treat for your family. It is less fuss if you heat several inches of oil in a small saucepan and fry in several batches rather than using lots of oil and a large container.

GLAZING is very similar to boiling except that when the onions are almost crisp-tender, add 1 tablespoon sugar, 1 tablespoon unsalted butter, and freshly milled black pepper to taste. Reduce the heat to low and cook, uncovered, until all but a few tablespoons of the liquid has boiled away. Stir or shake the pan so the onions are coated in the syrup produced and start to brown slightly.

ROASTING concentrates the flavor of onions and garlic. Just peel onions (cut them in wedges, if they are large) or garlic cloves and toss them with oil, salt and freshly milled black pepper to taste, and herbs, if you want. Spread them out in a roasting pan and put them in the oven. You can use any temperature you wish, so they are the perfect accompaniment to roasted meats and other roasted vegetables. But if you are doing them alone, try 400°F for 20 to 45 minutes, depending upon size. Either way, give them a stir and check for doneness every 10 to 12 minutes.

SAUTÉING really brings out the flavor of onions. Sautéed onions are the perfect accompaniment, topping, or garnish for meat, fish, pasta, rice, and other

Having a Good Cry?

When you cut open the cells of an onion, you release both a volatile sulfuric compound and an enzyme that cooperate to produce the eye-irritating substance propenylsulfenic acid. Fortunately, it decomposes rapidly and is also destroyed by cooking, so your eyes recover quickly. But it causes enough annoyance that almost every cook has a remedy. Here are some we have been told:

- Chill the onions in the refrigerator or freezer before cutting.
- Peel the onions under water.
- Put vinegar on the cutting board before cutting the onions.
- Keep a gas flame or candle burning beside your cutting board.
- Wear goggles.

vegetables. Just slice or chop the onions and cook them in a heavy skillet over medium heat with enough butter or oil to make them glisten. Stir them constantly until they reach the texture you like. Onions contain so much natural sugar that long, low-temperature cooking without liquid causes them to caramelize to a delicious golden brown. The high sugar content is also what makes it easy to burn them if you don't keep a careful watch.

STIR-FRYING is a natural for alliums. They are the ideal way to start almost any stir-fry combination. And, once they are in the pan, a flavorful dish is assured.

Preserving

Because of the availability of storage onions, freezing onions is not something people often think of doing. However, if your CSA has an abundant crop, you may want to take advantage of this option. Onions freeze well, and it is very convenient to have containers of them in your freezer peeled, sliced, or chopped and ready to use in any cooked dish. To prepare small onions for freezing whole, blanch them until heated through, then peel and pack them in freezer containers. To freeze slices, peel and slice the onions, then blanch, pack, and freeze. To freeze chopped onions, peel, quarter, and blanch, then cool, chop, and freeze. Chopped green onions may be frozen, but we don't recommend freezing whole green onions because it toughens the greens, which is not noticeable when they are chopped. To use frozen onions, add them to simmering soups, stews, and sauces still frozen. To use them in baked products or stuffings, thaw them long enough to separate the pieces.

Alliums Are Good for You

Although all the onion family members are considered to be healthy as well as delicious additions to the diet, garlic has traditionally been singled out as a preventive measure. Just what is garlic supposed to be good for? Well, if your grandmother prescribed it to prevent colds, she wasn't the first to ascribe medicinal properties to garlic. Greek and Roman writers suggested it to cure a variety of problems ranging from lack of courage to rabies. This reputation (see Alternative Uses for Garlic, above) has been passed along from generation to generation right up to the present. Today, medical researchers take garlic seriously as a potential aid in strengthening the immune system and treating infections, heart disease, and cancer. All members of the onion family are low in calories, moderately good sources of fiber, virtually fat free, and high in vitamin C, potassium, and folic acid. A ½-cup serving of chopped boiled onions provides about 9 percent of your recommended daily allowance of vitamin C and 8 percent of folic acid.

MUSHROOM-GARLIC TRIANGLES

MAKES 18 TRIANGLES

This is the perfect showcase for homegrown garlic. When the garlic is ready to harvest, CSA members often go to the farm to help. The fresh garlic aroma in the field is intoxicating, and it is hard having to leave the delicate little heads to dry in a shed and wait the several weeks necessary for them to dry and be ready to use.

3 to 6 small garlic cloves, finely chopped
2 tablespoons olive oil
10 ounces white mushrooms, chopped
1 (3-ounce) package cream cheese, softened
Salt and freshly milled black pepper
1 (17.3-ounce) package frozen puff pastry (2 sheets), thawed

Sauté the garlic in the oil in a large skillet over medium heat until softened but not browned, about 1 minute. Add the mushrooms and sauté until soft and most of the liquid has evaporated. Turn the heat to low; add the cream cheese to the mixture in the skillet and stir until melted. Allow the mixture to cool slightly; taste and add salt and pepper.

Preheat the oven to 375°F. Line a rimmed baking sheet with aluminum foil.

Cut each puff pastry sheet lengthwise into 3 equal strips; cut each strip crosswise into 3 rectangles. Divide the mushroom mixture among the rectangles, placing a mound in the center of each. Moisten the edges of the pastry rectangles; fold each to form a triangle enclosing the filling. Pinch the edges to seal.

Arrange the triangles on the baking sheet. Bake for 12 to 15 minutes, until puffed and golden brown. Serve hot or at room temperature.

Garlic Greens

The garlic plant provides us with valuable ingredients well before it forms its bulbs. The first leaves that sprout when the cloves are planted have a mild garlic taste that adds plenty of flavor to soups and stews without overpowering them. If the leaves are pulled, the plant won't form bulbs; nevertheless, farmers often plant rows of garlic just to use as greens.

Hard-neck garlic varieties send up a scape (flower stem) that must be picked before it flowers. If it's left on the plant, the bulb won't be as large. So we can use the scape without sacrificing the bulb—we can have our garlic and eat it, too. Garlic scape can be chopped and added to salad dressings, sautéed for sauces and stews, and substituted for garlic wherever it's called for. Its taste is less harsh and less lasting, which is often a blessing.

ONION BISCUITS (TZIBELE KICHEL)

MAKES 45 BISCUITS

These delicious biscuits will bring the whole family to the kitchen as soon as they start to bake. If you have any left over after dinner, they will be good in lunch boxes the next day. It was submitted by Shirley Stein (with a little help from Mendy).

4 medium onions
3 large eggs
1 cup vegetable oil
3 tablespoons poppy seeds
1 teaspoon salt
½ teaspoon freshly milled black pepper
3 cups all-purpose flour
1 tablespoon baking powder

Preheat the oven to 375°F. Lightly grease 2 baking sheets. Coarsely grate the onions in a food processor.

Beat the eggs in a large bowl until fluffy. Beat in the oil, poppy seeds, salt, and pepper. Fold in the flour and baking powder until just combined, then fold in the grated onions.

Drop the soft dough by tablespoonful onto the baking sheets to make 45 biscuits. Bake the biscuits for 35 to 40 minutes, until browned.

CHÈVRE-ONION TOPPER

MAKES 6 TO 8 SERVINGS

Chef Jeff Nagel of Caprine Estates designed this recipe to showcase the Caprine Estates' plain *fromage de chèvre*. He uses all organic produce to complement the organic cheese produced at the estates' dairy.

5 ounces fresh chèvre (goat cheese)
1 tablespoon chopped fresh thyme, or
  1 teaspoon dried
2 garlic cloves, finely chopped

Salt and freshly milled white pepper
2 tablespoons olive oil
2 medium red onions, thinly sliced
1 tablespoon sugar

Combine the chèvre, thyme, and garlic in a small bowl. Add salt and white pepper to taste and mix well. Either form the chèvre into a shape of your choice (log or ball) or coat a wide shallow bowl with vegetable cooking spray or plastic wrap and firmly press the chèvre mixture into the bowl; cover and refrigerate for 30 minutes.

Heat the oil in a medium skillet over medium heat. Add the onions and cook, stirring occasionally, until they are translucent, 12 to 15 minutes. Sprinkle with the sugar and season with salt and white pepper. Mix well and continue to cook over medium heat until the onions deepen in color and caramelize, about 5 minutes.

Place the chèvre mixture on a serving platter; top with the caramelized onions, making sure to cover completely. Serve immediately with your choice of crackers or bread.

Just add a salad and you have a meal. Contributed by coeditor of this book, Joanne Hayes of the Carnegie Hill/Yorkville CSA in Manhattan, it is a convenient busy-evening supper because it can be left to bake while the cook does other things.

1 tablespoon unsalted butter	1 1/2 cups half-and-half
1 1/2 pounds yellow onions, thinly sliced	3 large eggs
1/3 cup dried couscous	1/2 teaspoon salt
2 cups grated Cheddar cheese	1/8 to 1/4 teaspoon ground red pepper

Preheat the oven to 350°F. Generously grease a 9-inch pie pan.

Heat the butter in a large, heavy skillet over medium-low heat. Add the onions and cook slowly, stirring occasionally, until they are golden and tender, about 20 minutes.

Sprinkle the couscous into the bottom of the pie pan. Transfer half of the onions onto the couscous and sprinkle with half of the cheese. Repeat.

Whisk the half-and-half, eggs, salt, and the desired amount of red pepper in a medium bowl until combined. Pour the egg mixture over the onions and cheese in the pie pan.

Bake for 25 to 30 minutes, until the surface is light brown and the center looks set. Let stand for 5 minutes; cut into 4 wedges and serve.

FRIED ONION AND CHEDDAR PIE

MAKES 4 SERVINGS

What's a Scallion?

There seems to be a lot of confusion about the true identity of scallions, and it's no wonder. The slim green alliums with underdeveloped bulbs that you find in your market by that name can be a number of things. If the white part is straight and there is a noticeable root end, it could be a baby leek, or if the base looks cut, it could be the top of a shallot. If the white base is slightly rounded, it is probably a baby onion or green onion. Scallions were named for the Mediterranean seaport Ascalon (now the Israeli city of Ashkelon); the term was used in early cookbooks for mature shallots as well. However, it doesn't really matter a lot in your kitchen which green allium you are using, because, although they vary slightly in flavor intensity, they are certainly interchangeable in recipes.

POTATO-LEEK SOUP WITH WILD GARLIC FLOWERS

SERVES 6

Naturalist Euell Gibbons called wild garlic (also known as ramp) "the sweetest and best of the wild onions." "Sweet" is a relative term, though, because ramp's scent is far from delicate. Wild garlic is native to most of the east coast of North America, but until recently (chefs have rediscovered ramp in the past decade), it was used only in rural areas of the South, where it's a much-loved delicacy and a harbinger of spring. Early settlers were introduced to ramps by Native Americans, who used it to spice up blander foods, as well as medicinally (modern scientists now concur that members of the onion family have healing properties). This recipe was contributed by Miriam Kresh, who notes that although the butter and sour cream are optional, they add a luxurious richness of texture and taste.

6 medium potatoes, peeled
Olive oil
1 large onion, sliced
1 large leek, cleaned and sliced
1 bay leaf
½ teaspoon dried thyme
2 cups milk

2 tablespoons all-purpose flour
1 cup sour cream (optional)
3 green onions, sliced
2 tablespoons dry white wine
2 tablespoons unsalted butter (optional)
Salt and freshly milled black pepper
6 wild garlic flower heads (optional)

Thinly slice the potatoes, then cut into 1-inch squares. Heat enough oil in a large soup pot to cover the bottom. Sauté the potatoes, stirring constantly to keep them from sticking to the bottom of the pot, until they are almost tender, 8 to 10 minutes. Add the sliced onion and leek. Sauté, stirring constantly, until the vegetables are golden, about 5 minutes.

Add 4 cups water, the bay leaf, and the thyme and cook until the vegetables are quite soft, about 20 minutes. In a cup or small bowl, mix a little of the milk into the flour until smooth. Whisk it thoroughly into the soup, then add the rest of the milk. Bring just to a boil, stirring constantly until thickened.

When the soup is heated through, remove the bay leaf. Stir in the sour cream, if using, the green onions, the wine, and the butter, if using. Continue to heat but do not allow the soup to boil again. Add salt and pepper to taste. Add the garlic flowers, if using, and stir just until they have wilted. Serve immediately.

Garlic Bread

Nothing is as enticing as the aroma of garlic bread toasting in the oven just as dinner is ready. And it is so easy to make. For a classic presentation, just split a loaf of fresh Italian bread and place the halves, cut side up, on a baking sheet. For ease in serving, make diagonal cuts down to about ¾ inch from the crust on each half. Spread the cut surfaces with softened unsalted butter; sprinkle them with finely chopped CSA garlic (or whatever you have) to taste, 2 tablespoons grated Parmesan, and a dusting of paprika. Toast the bread in a 375°F oven for 5 to 7 minutes, until the edges begin to brown. A little finely chopped fresh parsley, basil, oregano, thyme, or rosemary over the garlic can provide variations on the theme, as can using rolls, English muffins, or thick slices of bread in place of the Italian loaf.

FRESH GREEN GARLIC AND LEEKS WITH PASTA AND OLIVES

MAKES 4 SERVINGS

Stephenie Caughlin, owner and manager of Seabreeze Organic Farm, located in Del Mar, California, gave up teaching to commit herself to 100 percent natural production of produce, herbs, and flowers. She says her farm "is the dream come true that I bring to people's doors every day. I don't know a better way to live." This is a great recipe that takes less than a half hour to make.

8 ounces spaghetti
Salt
4 to 8 cups tatsoi leaves, to taste
6 green garlic stems
6 medium leeks, cleaned
2 tablespoons olive oil
1 cup sliced green olives
Pinch of hot red pepper flakes

Cook the spaghetti in boiling salted water according to the package directions. Meanwhile, thoroughly wash the tatsoi leaves and remove the stems if they are tough. Remove and chop the white bulbs of the garlic and leeks; wrap and refrigerate the green tops to make stock or for another use.

Heat the oil in a large, heavy saucepan over medium heat. Add the tatsoi, garlic, and leeks. Sauté for about 2 minutes. Add the olives, salt to taste, and the red pepper flakes. Sauté for another minute. Toss with the cooked spaghetti and serve.

LENTIL-LEEK BURRITOS

MAKES 4 SERVINGS

Marjo M. van Patten, a member of Bluebird Hills Farm in Springfield, Ohio, loves being forced to be creative in the kitchen. She says that every week's share is like a potluck, requiring her to find new ways to use old and new ingredients. These easy-to-make burritos are a good way to introduce children (and adults) to leeks.

2 small leeks, cleaned and finely
   chopped
3/4 teaspoon dried oregano
3/4 teaspoon chili powder
1/2 teaspoon paprika
1/2 teaspoon hot red pepper sauce,
   or to taste

1/2 teaspoon ground cumin
2 cups cooked lentils
4 large flour tortillas
2 tablespoons grated low-fat cheese
4 tomatoes, quartered
1 tablespoon lime juice
2 green onions, finely chopped

Lightly coat a large skillet with vegetable cooking spray. Add the leeks, oregano, chili powder, paprika, hot red pepper sauce, and cumin. Sauté over medium heat until the mixture is fragrant and the leeks are just tender, 5 to 6 minutes. Mix in the lentils.

Divide the lentil mixture among the tortillas, spreading it along one edge of each. Sprinkle with the cheese and roll up to form burritos.

Wipe out the frying pan and respray. Place the burritos in the pan, seam side down. Heat on medium-high until the bottoms of the burritos are just browned, about 2 minutes.

Meanwhile, in a food processor or blender, combine the tomatoes and lime juice. Process briefly until the tomatoes are coarsely chopped. (Coarsely chopping the tomatoes by hand and adding the lime juice also works.)

Flip the burritos and pour the tomato mixture over them, cover loosely, and simmer until heated through, about 4 minutes. Sprinkle with the green onions and serve hot.

Chef Ric Orlando, who calls himself "a deliciously opinionated" chef, and his staff at New World Home Cooking, near Woodstock, New York, have made a strong commitment to keeping the majority of their inventory sustainable and organic. They've forged relationships with local produce and livestock farms in the Hudson Valley so that their menus can include healthy vegetables and meats. Ric is host of *Ric's TV Kitchen,* a public-television show that features clean food. This recipe uses a lot of mellow roasted garlic, is easy and affordable to make, and is a great alternative to potatoes, rice, or pasta. Serve it as a side dish to hearty meat, game, or poultry dishes.

24 garlic cloves, unpeeled
Olive oil
Salt and freshly milled black pepper
8 cups 1-inch cubes fresh Italian or
    French bread
5 large eggs
2 cups milk
2 cups heavy cream

⅓ cup grated Romano cheese
2 tablespoons bourbon or brandy
    (optional)
1 teaspoon chopped fresh thyme, or a
    slightly rounded ¼ teaspoon dried
1 teaspoon chopped fresh rosemary,
    or a slightly rounded ¼ teaspoon
    dried

Preheat the oven to 425°F. Snip off and discard the tip from each garlic clove; toss the cloves with 1 tablespoon olive oil, and salt and pepper to taste. Spread out on a rimmed baking sheet and bake for 20 to 30 minutes, until softened. Let cool to the touch and gently peel.

Meanwhile, generously grease a 13- by 9-inch baking pan or dish with olive oil. Arrange the bread evenly in the pan.

Mash the garlic cloves with a fork in a large bowl. Add the eggs and beat until slightly fluffy. Beat in the milk, cream, cheese, bourbon, if using, thyme, rosemary, ½ teaspoon salt, and pepper to taste. Pour the mixture evenly over the bread.

Bake for 40 to 50 minutes, or until the top is golden brown, and serve hot.

LUSTROUS LEEKS

MAKES 6 SERVINGS

This recipe was submitted by Farm Fresh to You CSA, which is located in the Capay Valley, nestled in the Coastal Range fifty miles west of Sacramento. The hot summers and cold winters of the valley result in kissed-by-the-sun summer and robust winter produce. The Capay Valley is chockful of safe, responsible farms, serving the Sacramento and San Francisco areas.

3 large leeks
1 tablespoon white wine vinegar
2 tablespoons extra-virgin olive oil

1 medium tomato, quartered
2 tablespoons oil-cured black olives
1 1/2 tablespoons chopped fresh parsley

Trim the leek greens in a V to within 3 inches of the white bulb, leaving the roots intact. Split the leeks lengthwise. To remove the dirt, soak the leeks in a bowl of water to cover plus the white wine vinegar for 30 minutes. Rinse the leeks well under cold running water.

Cook the leeks in boiling salted water until tender, about 8 minutes. Drain well; cut off the roots and pat dry.

Heat the oil in a medium skillet. Add the leeks and cook until golden. Stir in the tomato, olives, and parsley; cover, and cook until the tomatoes are just heated through. Transfer the leeks to a serving platter; spoon the tomato mixture over the top. Let cool to room temperature and serve, or cover and refrigerate to serve cold.

Meet the Farmers

Pauline Lord and David Harlow
White Gate Farm, East Lyme, Connecticut

Pauline and David lived utterly different lives before arriving at White Gate Farm. Pauline, fifty-two, was working as a psychotherapist and her husband, David, fifty-six, was a geophysicist. The two, who were living in Southern California when they decided it was time for a change, had long envisioned farming in their future. They saw opportunity in a one-hundred-acre former dairy farm that Pauline's parents had bought when Pauline was in her twenties. Pauline's mother had been urging them to move back for some time, so they tried out farming for one summer, explored the market, and adored it. They have been certified organic for three years. In 2002, their first season as a CSA, the farm had forty members.

What made the concept of small-farm life important enough for them to uproot their lives? The farm and the CSA concept respond to a lot of their values, Pauline says. "My husband and I really care about protecting the soil, saving the space, and preserving the farmland." It disturbs Pauline that Americans spend a much smaller percentage of their money on food than do people in other developed countries. "Good food is quite expensive to grow," she says. "It would be helpful if people got out of the mind-set of expecting cheap produce. Also, farming is a lot more complex than people realize. The image of the farmer has been dumbed down in the popular mind, but farmers are really required to be skillful, intelligent people. You make lots of decisions every day and there's always a great variety of things to do." Pauline likes the diversity. One day she's marketing and the next day she'll be in the fields weeding. She says, "It's a good balance."

CHAPTER SIX

STALKS AND STEMS

This small chapter holds some unusual produce items that have very little to do with one another except that they are sturdy stems or aboveground roots that serve the purpose of stems. With the exception of asparagus and celery, they are all specialties that are more likely to show up in a CSA share than in the local market. Asparagus, cardoons, celery, fennel, and rhubarb all serve as the supporting structure of a plant. Their function of conducting food and water between the roots and leaves of a plant makes them crisp, juicy, and flavorful additions to any menu.

Asparagus officinalis is a remarkable perennial vegetable of the Liliaceae family. Its green or blanched-white stems function as leaves and the leaves are reduced to scales, while the stalks of its parent plant produce fluffy whisks of fernlike greens. Although its origin is not known, asparagus has been cultivated in the eastern Mediterranean for more than two thousand years and appears by that name in Roman writings. In ancient times, asparagus was cultivated more for medicinal than culinary use. It was prescribed to relieve toothache and prevent bee stings.

Cardoons are long celerylike stalks with a narrow top leaf. Botanically *Cynara cardunculus,* the plant is a member of the daisy (Asteraceae) family, and a close relative of the artichoke (*Cynara scolymus*). It is variously reported as either the precursor to or the derivative of the globe artichoke. A favorite with the early Greeks and Romans and during medieval times, it had slipped from use in northern Europe by the early nineteenth century. Spanish colonists introduced it into South America and it now grows wild there.

Celery, *Apium graveolens,* is probably native to the Mediterranean and was used wild for many centuries before it was cultivated in Italy and northern

Europe for use as an herbal medicine. Its use as a flavoring element in cooking was first recorded in the seventeenth century. Both wild and cultivated celery were brought to America and planted in colonial gardens. However, the climate of California was more suited to celery's needs, and commercial production became centered there. In the late nineteenth century, when the transcontinental railroad was first able to bring vegetables from California's farms to the East, top restaurants sold several stalks of celery as an appetizer at prices similar to those of caviar. Glassware companies of the era designed special celery goblets in which to serve the premium product.

Fennel, *Foeniculum vulgare,* is mentioned as a seasoning in classical Greek and Roman writings and was probably used around the Mediterranean long before. Early types of fennel, bitter and sweet, are used mostly for flavoring; dried stalks, for grilling and to produce seeds. The vegetable finocchio, or Florence fennel, was probably not developed until the seventeenth century and was brought to America by Italian immigrants. Until the past decade, it was only available in ethnic markets, but now has become a popular fall vegetable on restaurant menus. Hopefully markets will soon stop labeling it "anise," which is an entirely different plant.

Rhubarb consists of several species of the genus *Rheum* and members of the buckwheat, or Polygonaceae, family. Native to the cooler areas of Asia, rhubarb was used medicinally in China, and the dried stems were being exported to Greece and Rome by the first century C.E. The pungent oxalic-acid-containing stalks were probably not used in cooking until sugar was readily available. English recipes did not start appearing until the early nineteenth century. In America, it became known as pie plant because of its most common use. Rhubarb leaves and roots have so much oxalic acid that they are toxic and should be discarded.

An asparagus bed is an investment in the future. Although it can take three to four years to be productive, a well-maintained bed can last for years. There are both dark and light green varieties. Dark green asparagus arrive early in the season and are harvested when the stems are about 8 inches out of the ground. The same variety may be planted in trenches and gradually covered with soil as it grows to produce the blanched, or white, asparagus that is pop-

In the Field

ular in Europe. Light green varieties tend to appear several weeks later. To maintain flavor, asparagus should quickly be chilled after harvesting.

Cardoons, which are ready for harvest in about 120 days, are much easier to grow than artichokes, which sometimes take up to six months for the edible flowers to appear. They have adapted to the California climate so well that they grow wild and are considered weeds in some areas. They should be harvested while the shank is still small so they will be tender.

It is difficult to grow celery and get the wide, solid stems and compact bunches that we consider good quality; it must be grown under near-greenhouse conditions with even moisture and temperature. There are two distinct types of celery, 'Golden Heart,' which is bleached white, and 'Pascal,' which is light to dark green; Pascal is the more popular because it has been bred to be less stringy. A third type, cutting celery, which grows well in most regions, doesn't provide juicy, crisp stalks, but its leaves and stems are loaded with celery flavor and are valuable additions to soups and stews.

Fennel bulbs need cool weather to develop properly; the plants put out graceful, wispy fronds in late summer but do not grow voluptuous, juicy bulbs until early fall. They do not last long once out of the ground, so it is best to harvest a little at a time until frost threatens and then to remove all that remains, as the fragile bulbs are high in moisture and freeze easily.

From early spring until the first frost, rhubarb will put out new growth whenever you harvest it; the first harvest is always the most abundant, though, which is why we associate rhubarb with spring. Plants with pale green stems more closely resemble the original variety, while the rosy to cherry red versions are later developments. Both are equally delicious when cooked. The hardy plants survive for years and require very little care, but they do need some cold weather to encourage winter dormancy, so it's difficult to grow rhubarb in warm climates.

Selecting the Best

When selecting asparagus, look for stalks that are straight and fresh-looking. They should be crisp, yet tender, with compact pointed tips. Avoid wilted stalks, loose or damp heads, and woody bottoms. Since the exterior of asparagus stalks may be stringy, fat stalks will be more tender, because they have a larger moist, stringless interior.

Cardoons are more tender when they are young and small. The leaves should be very dark green and the stalks should be crisp. As they age, the outer portion will become tough and woody and may have to be discarded.

Select a head of celery that is crisp and heavy. The leaves should be fresh-looking and the stalks should be brittle enough to snap easily. Avoid brown or cracked outer stems. Stalks of medium length and thickness will be more tender and mild than longer, wider ones. The inside of the stem should be smooth, not rough or puffy, or the celery may be hollow. If you can get to it to see, a crisp, pale heart indicates good celery.

Fennel is very perishable and should be used as close to harvest as possible. Look for small lustrous bulbs and avoid any that look dry, brown, or cracked, or have moist patches. The bulbs will become more fibrous and less flavorful with storage. Select fennel that still has the tops, as they make good garnishes.

Rhubarb perfection is very much like that of the other stalks. It should be straight and crisp, without brown or black spots, splits, or bare patches. Rhubarb leaves are poisonous because of their high oxalic-acid content, so you might as well have them removed before you take them home. If purchasing rhubarb by weight, select stems that have all of the leaf removed.

After You Pick Up or Buy

Because of their high water content, all the stalks and stems must be kept in such a way as to avoid dehydration. It is important not only to keep them tightly covered, but to give them a source of moisture at the root end.

Asparagus loses flavor and crispness rapidly if it gets warm. It is important to store it in the coolest part of the refrigerator and to use it as soon as possible. Asparagus will maintain its quality best if the bottoms are trimmed and the bunch is placed, standing up, in water in a mug, glass, or measuring cup.

Cardoons should be kept somewhere cool and used as soon as possible. If storing them in the refrigerator, you might first want to trim off and discard any woody outer portions to save space.

Celery must be stored, well wrapped, in the refrigerator to keep it crisp. Actually, if you had the room, the ideal way to store celery would be as you do asparagus, upright in a container of water.

Fennel bulbs should have the stalks/greens removed before storage so that they will not continue to use nutrients from the bulb. Wrap both tightly and refrigerate until ready to use.

Rhubarb is the least fragile of these stalks and stems. You can keep it in the refrigerator crisper in an open plastic bag for several days.

Preparing Uncooked

Although rarely done, asparagus can be served raw. It is best to select young, tender stalks that have been freshly harvested so that their skins have not dried out and toughened. Remove the root end as far up as it is woody, or peel the bottom third and remove only the portion that is not tender. Remove the tiny leaves and slice the stalk thinly crosswise. Add the asparagus slices to a baby-lettuce salad or see Asparagus Soup with White Truffle "Sour Cream" (page 108).

Celery is a natural for raw consumption. In fact, much more celery is eaten raw than cooked. Thoroughly rinse celery stalks or scrub with a vegetable brush. Trim off the tops (and save them for soup or stock) and the root ends (you can discard these), and slice the stalks diagonally crosswise or chop them to add to salads. Cut into sticks for snacks and crudités.

Fennel is a sweet and crunchy addition to a salad or crudité plate. Or it can be dipped into *bagna cauda,* fondue, or herbed cream cheese or sour cream dips. Scrub the outer layers with a vegetable brush and cold water. Remove the strings if it seems fibrous, trim off the roots leaving the root end intact so the slices will hold together, and slice the bulb into thin wedges that are attached at the bottom.

Cardoons and rhubarb are not used uncooked.

Preparing Cooked

Asparagus is the most fragile of these stems and stalks and should be cooked as little as possible. Trim and clean the asparagus as directed in "Preparing Uncooked" above. You can use larger, thicker stalks for cooking than for eating raw. The old rule of snapping off the asparagus stem as close to the bottom as it breaks off easily can be stretched a little if you peel the bottom of the stem with a vegetable peeler and then test it to see where it becomes tough. As long as you are using a vegetable peeler, nip off the tiny leaves as well. This will surely give you an extra inch of asparagus to enjoy. Asparagus may be blanched before using cold in salads and crudités. It can be boiled, broiled or grilled, deep-fried, microwaved, roasted, sautéed, steamed, and stir-fried. Just be sure to keep it brief.

Cardoons should always be cooked. To prepare them, remove the outer stems, as they never become tender when cooked. Split the head in half lengthwise and peel as much of the inside and outer skin as you can get to. Cut them into 2- to 3-inch pieces and boil them in acidulated water to cover. (Use 1 teaspoon lemon juice or vinegar per cup of water.) Depending upon the maturity of the cardoons, they should be crisp-tender in 15 to 20 minutes. Once cooked, serve them in a mix of fall vegetables or as a dipper for *bagna cauda,* or puree them for soup.

Cooked celery is a quiet addition to soups, stews, and stir-fries. Small heads of celery, quartered, can be braised as an accompaniment to roasts. To cook celery, clean and trim the head as directed in "Preparing Uncooked." Celery cooks very quickly. Chopped pieces should be simmered only 6 to 8 minutes and single stalks 10 to 12. Sautéed and stir-fried, celery can take even less time.

Fennel should be cleaned and trimmed as directed in "Preparing Uncooked," then cut into ½- to 1-inch wedges and simmered or braised just until crisp-tender, 20 to 25 minutes. Fennel puree pairs well with carrot puree or mashed potato. Thin wedges of fennel may be deep-fried for a delicious garnish on just about anything.

Rhubarb should be trimmed below the leaf, and any sign of leaf or root should be discarded, as they are poisonous due to their high oxalic-acid content. The root end should be discarded to the point where it becomes straight. The remaining stalk should be thoroughly rinsed in cool water and cut into 1-inch or smaller pieces to be used in recipes such as Rhubarb Sauce (page 112), rhubarb pie, and The Church Potluck Rhubarb Cake (page 114).

Preserving

Because of their high water content, stalks and stems are not usually good candidates for freezing. Asparagus freezes well but must be blanched and thoroughly drained before packing. Fully cooked cardoons and blanched rhubarb may be frozen but are quite watery once thawed. Rhubarb sauce freezes well and makes a delicious dessert sauce if processed and served while still frozen. These three kinds of stalks and stems could be canned, but they keep their texture and flavor better when frozen.

Celery and fennel should not be frozen; the tasteless, stringy puddle that results from freezing either of them is very disappointing. Both celery and fennel can be pickled with good results.

Stalks and Stems Are Good for You

Because they contain a lot of moisture, stalks and stems can provide a satisfying serving with little fat and few calories. In addition, asparagus is high in potassium and vitamins A and C, and low in sodium. Although a bit higher in sodium, cardoons are also high in potassium and a decent source of calcium. Celery and fennel are good sources of potassium and so low in calories that you barely need to count them. Ditto for rhubarb, except that it really needs to be paired with a lot of sugar to become tasty and that's where the calories come in.

CELERY STALKS WITH GINGER TOFU DIP

MAKES 1¾ CUPS, ABOUT 8 SERVINGS

Bill Enkhausen and Peter Fleury farm at Oasis Garden, nine acres of pesticide- and chemical-free land with an average soil depth of twelve feet (yes, feet). When they speak about the dirt at their east Austin farm, they sound like they're describing something wonderful and delicious. This recipe was submitted by one of their members.

1 pound soft tofu
¼ cup sliced green onion
2 tablespoons soy sauce
1 tablespoon finely chopped peeled fresh ginger
1 tablespoon toasted sesame oil
1 garlic clove, finely chopped
¼ teaspoon ground red pepper
6 cups quartered celery stalks, or other raw vegetables such as cucumber slices, carrot sticks, red or green bell pepper strips, sugar snap peas, or cherry tomatoes

Rinse the tofu under cool running water, let drain, then combine in a food processor or blender with the green onion, soy sauce, ginger, sesame oil, garlic, and red pepper until smooth. Pour into a small bowl; accompany with the celery stalks or other raw vegetables.

Until Steve Waxman of the Carnegie Hill/Yorkville CSA in Manhattan contributed this recipe to the group's newsletter, members weren't quite sure what to do with the beautiful fennel that arrived as the weather got cool. Now they simply wish it would arrive more often.

1 large or 2 small fennel bulbs	*½ teaspoon ground ginger*
2 tablespoons olive oil	*2 cups or more vegetable stock*
1 medium carrot, chopped	*1 (28-ounce) can whole tomatoes*
1 small onion, chopped	*Salt and freshly milled black pepper*
1 garlic clove, finely chopped	*Dry mustard*

Cut the fennel into slivers, reserving the tops. Heat the oil in a skillet; add the fennel, carrot, onion, garlic, and ginger. Sauté until the onion begins to color, about 4 minutes. Add 1 cup of the stock and simmer until the fennel and carrot begin to soften. If the stock cooks out, add more.

Add the tomatoes and another cup of stock. Season with salt and pepper and mustard to taste. Cook until everything is tender enough so that it will blend well. Blend the mixture in small batches; return to the saucepan and heat. Serve with sprigs of the reserved fennel tops as garnish.

TOMATO-FENNEL SOUP

MAKES 4 SERVINGS

ASPARAGUS SOUP WITH WHITE TRUFFLE "SOUR CREAM"

MAKES 6 SERVINGS

Roxanne Klein, chef/owner of Roxanne's in Larkspur, California, told us that for this recipe, "we handpick the sweetest, most incredible-tasting asparagus from our local farmers' market and our own garden. Fresh-picked spinach and herbs add some balance." Roxanne's is a 100 percent organic, living-foods restaurant. Nothing served in the restaurant is heated beyond 115°F, which means that it is essential to have the very best produce.

White Truffle "Sour Cream"
 (recipe follows)
2 cups firmly packed torn spinach
 leaves with stems
1 ripe avocado, peeled and pitted
½ cup chopped asparagus stems
 (no tips)
¼ cup chopped peeled celery
¼ cup Nama Shoyu (see Note)

2½ tablespoons lemon juice
4 teaspoons chopped green onion
2 fresh thyme sprigs
1 tablespoon chopped fresh tarragon
2 teaspoons finely chopped garlic
2 teaspoons salt
⅛ teaspoon freshly milled black
 pepper
⅛ teaspoon ground red pepper

Bagna Cauda

The quintessential dip for cardoons, celery, or fennel, this recipe instantly becomes a favorite of most people who try it. It's not just that it's delicious and can be made in no time flat; it also scents the kitchen with a heady aroma of garlic and anchovy and pulls any crowd together as they gather around it. Heat ½ cup good-quality olive oil and 4 tablespoons unsalted butter in a saucepan. Add 6 to 8 minced fresh garlic cloves and simmer until the garlic is very soft, about 10 minutes. Add 4 to 6 anchovy fillets and continue cooking until they fall apart, about another 5 minutes. Mash the garlic and anchovies until they all but disappear (you can also whirl the mixture in a food processor or blender for a few minutes). Some people add a tablespoon or two of heavy cream. If you can, place the *bagna* on a hot plate, so that it stays warm throughout the evening. Serve it with chunks of vegetable—cardoon is the traditional accompaniment, but celery, fennel, blanched asparagus, and some cubes of the best bread you can find are easy substitutes. Other options include carrot sticks, green pepper strips, squash spears, and cherry tomatoes. It will keep in the refrigerator, in a tightly covered jar, for several days.

A day ahead, start the White Truffle "Sour Cream."

Just before serving, working in two batches, puree 3 cups water and the spinach, avocado, asparagus, celery, Nama Shoyu, lemon juice, green onion, thyme, tarragon, garlic, salt, black pepper, and red pepper in a blender until smooth. Pass through a fine strainer.

Divide the soup among 6 bowls and garnish with White Truffle "Sour Cream."

NOTE: Nama Shoyu is an aged, nonpasteurized soy sauce. If you can't find it, use a good-quality organic soy sauce.

WHITE TRUFFLE "SOUR CREAM": Combine ¾ cup Thai coconut meat (see Note), ⅓ cup raw cashews that have been soaked for 10 to 12 hours in filtered water, 3 tablespoons extra-virgin olive oil, 2 tablespoons lemon juice, 2 tablespoons water, 1 teaspoon honey-date paste or honey, and ½ teaspoon Celtic or sea salt in a food processor or blender and process until smooth. Stir in ½ teaspoon white truffle oil; set aside.

NOTE: A Thai, or green, coconut is an immature coconut in which the interior is soft and custardlike. To prepare the coconut, poke a hole in the pointy end with a steel knife or a clean screwdriver. Drain out the coconut water. Cut the coconut in half with a cleaver (start at the top, then work down one side until you can break it open and separate the halves), and rinse out the inside of each half. Use a spoon to scoop out the meat. Trim off any brown bits; dice and measure ¾ cup.

GRILLED ASPARAGUS WITH SUMMER VEGETABLES AND SPICY YOGURT SAUCE

MAKES 4 SERVINGS

Vince Alberici, executive chef at the Marker Restaurant in Philadelphia's Adam's Mark Hotel, contributed this enticing summer appetizer. Vince developed a relationship with Branch Creek Farms in nearby Bucks County, Pennsylvania, after being "blown away" by the intense flavors of their organic vegetables and lettuces at a tasting dinner some twelve years ago. "You're eating the essence of the vegetable when it's at its zenith going from the ground to the plate and into your mouth," says Vince, who buys vegetables from Branch Creek about twice a week. He likes serving this asparagus dish in the spring, when the local crop is at its peak.

Spicy Yogurt Sauce (recipe follows)
1 medium red bell pepper, quartered
1 medium yellow bell pepper, quartered
1 medium zucchini, cut into 12 slices
20 medium asparagus spears
3 tablespoons olive oil
Salt and freshly milled black pepper

Prepare the Spicy Yogurt Sauce. Preheat a charcoal grill or the broiler.

Rub the peppers, zucchini, and asparagus lightly with the oil. Place the peppers on the grill with the skin toward the heat source and grill until blackened. Remove and wrap in aluminum foil; set aside until cool enough to handle, then remove the skin.

Grill the zucchini for 2 minutes on each side and the asparagus for 1½ minutes on each side. Season the vegetables with salt and pepper to taste.

To serve, fan 3 zucchini slices at the top of each plate and arrange 5 asparagus spears in the center of the plate with red and yellow peppers on either side. Drizzle yogurt sauce over the vegetables.

SPICY YOGURT SAUCE: In a small skillet, sauté 1 seeded and chopped jalapeño pepper, 1 finely chopped garlic clove, and ½ teaspoon ground coriander in 3 tablespoons olive oil until the vegetables are softened but not browned, about 45 seconds. Combine the mixture with ½ cup plain low-fat yogurt, 2 finely chopped green onions, 2 tablespoons lemon juice, and salt and pepper to taste in a small bowl.

How does a CSA get started? Sometimes, the farmer does all the work of recruiting members and setting up deliveries or pickups. Other times, the farmer gets a little help. . . . On the Upper East Side of Manhattan, a group of six women, led by environmental activist Bonnie Lane Webber, set out to find a farmer and start the CSA that Bonnie knew the neighborhood needed and wanted. Though the meals she makes are always extraordinary, she likes to keep things simple, and this Asparagus Strata fits the bill. It can be made the night before it's eaten, and simply placed in the oven an hour before serving. Any vegetables, meats, and cheeses can be substituted for the ones listed.

ASPARAGUS STRATA

MAKES 6 SERVINGS

6 to 8 slices rye or whole wheat bread
1 pound bulk hot Italian sausage
  (or remove skins from links)
1/4 cup chopped onion
1/4 cup chopped bell pepper
1 tablespoon chopped garlic
1 pound asparagus, rinsed, trimmed,
  and cut into 1-inch pieces
8 large eggs

3 tablespoons all-purpose flour
2 tablespoons Dijon-style or other
  mustard
1 tablespoon Worcestershire sauce
Dash of hot red pepper sauce
3 cups whole milk
4 cups grated extra sharp Cheddar
  cheese (about 1 1/3 pounds)

Grease a 13- by 9-inch baking dish and line the bottom with bread.

Sauté the crumbled sausage in a large skillet over medium heat until it begins to brown. Add the onion, pepper, and garlic and sauté in the fat released by the sausage until the onion is browned and the sausage is cooked through.

Add the asparagus and cook 2 minutes.

Meanwhile, beat the eggs until fluffy; beat in the flour, mustard, Worcestershire sauce, and hot pepper sauce. Gradually beat in the milk. Sprinkle the sausage mixture over the bread in the baking dish; top with the cheese. Pour the egg mixture over all. Cover and let sit overnight in the refrigerator. (The strata can also be assembled and frozen until several hours before you are ready to bake it. Be sure to allow enough time for it to defrost.)

At least 1 hour before you want to serve, preheat the oven to 350°F. Bake the strata 45 to 60 minutes, or until it is just firm in the center. Cut into 6 rectangles and serve. Any leftovers can be frozen.

Rhubarb Sauce

Bring 2 pounds rhubarb, trimmed, rinsed, and cut into 1-inch pieces, and ¼ cup water to a boil in a large, heavy saucepan over low heat. Cover and cook, stirring frequently, until the rhubarb is very tender, 10 to 12 minutes. Stir in ¾ to 1 cup sugar, to taste, and ⅛ teaspoon salt; cook, stirring constantly, just until the sugar is dissolved, 3 to 4 minutes. Transfer to a serving bowl and set aside to cool to room temperature. Cover tightly and store in the refrigerator. Makes 4 cups.

Rhubarb Variations:
- Add 2 tablespoons finely chopped crystallized ginger, 2 teaspoons ground ginger, 1 teaspoon ground cinnamon, or ⅛ teaspoon ground cloves with the sugar.
- Add ½ cup sautéed chopped onions and ¼ cup dark raisins with the rhubarb to make rhubarb chutney.
- Cook 1 large apple or pear, peeled, quartered, and sliced crosswise, with the rhubarb.
- Fold 1 cup sliced fresh strawberries into the sauce once it has been cooked.

MARINATED FENNEL AND MUSHROOMS

MAKES 4 SERVINGS

For over twenty years, Tom Denison and Elizabeth Kerle of Denison Farms in Corvallis, Oregon, have been growing produce and selling direct to Oregon consumers. Tom says, "It feels good! In this fragmented world, it is healthy to build relationships, particularly around something as wholesome as real food." This recipe for fennel salad comes from Beaverton, Oregon, members Celeste and Rich Crimi. It takes just ten minutes to prepare. For a variation, they suggest adding ¼ to ½ teaspoon Dijon mustard to the dressing.

1 large fennel bulb
8 ounces white mushrooms
3 tablespoons olive oil
1½ tablespoons lemon juice

1 garlic clove, finely chopped
¼ cup finely chopped fresh dill
Salt and freshly milled black pepper

Remove the coarse outer stalks, root end, and leaves from the fennel; rinse and drain the fennel bulb. Cut the fennel bulb and the mushrooms into ⅛-inch-thick slices.

Whisk together the oil, lemon juice, and garlic in a large bowl until thick and yellow. Add the fennel, mushrooms, and dill; toss to combine. Season with salt and pepper to taste. Chill for at least 2 hours before serving, stirring occasionally.

Amy and Scott Richards and their four children moved to Oak Harbor, Washington, in the fall of 2000 to begin farming. The whole family is committed to closing the gap between farmers and consumers, and they supplement their shareholders' bounty by purchasing additional items from other farmers in their area.

BRAISED CELERY

MAKES 4 SERVINGS

1 head celery
3 bacon slices, quartered,
   or 2 tablespoons unsalted butter
1 medium onion, coarsely chopped

¾ cup vegetable stock
1 tablespoon chopped fresh parsley,
   or 1 teaspoon dried
Salt and freshly milled black pepper

Preheat the oven to 350°F. Rinse, drain, and trim the celery; cut the stalks into 2-inch pieces.

Sauté the bacon in a large, heavy ovenproof skillet for 4 to 5 minutes, until it begins to brown. (Or melt the butter.) Add the celery and onion and sauté until the onion begins to brown, 3 to 4 minutes.

Pour the stock over the mixture. Cover the skillet with an ovenproof lid or aluminum foil and braise the vegetables in the oven for 20 to 25 minutes, until the celery is tender. Stir in the parsley; season with salt and pepper to taste and serve.

THE CHURCH POTLUCK RHUBARB CAKE

MAKES 12 SERVINGS

The first time farmer Debby Kavakos of Stoneledge Farm, South Cairo, New York, gave rhubarb to her CSA members, she was surprised to find out that many of them had never seen it before. The next week, she printed the following recipe in her newsletter. Her mother had gotten it from a woman named Marge, who had brought the cake to every potluck dinner in their upstate New York church. Everyone remembers Marge for her rhubarb cake! The moist interior and crisp sugary crust are unforgettable.

TOPPING

1 cup chopped nuts
½ cup granulated sugar

2 tablespoons unsalted butter, melted
1 teaspoon ground cinnamon

CAKE

1 ½ cups packed light brown sugar
4 tablespoons unsalted butter, softened
1 large egg
1 cup plain low-fat yogurt
2 cups all-purpose flour

1 teaspoon baking soda
½ teaspoon salt
1 pound rhubarb, cut into 1-inch
    chunks

Preheat the oven to 350°F. Grease a 13- by 9-inch baking pan.

For the topping, combine the nuts, granulated sugar, melted butter, and cinnamon in a small bowl; set aside.

For the cake, beat the brown sugar, softened butter, and egg with an electric mixer until well blended; beat in the yogurt. Add the flour, baking soda, and salt to the butter mixture; stir to blend. Fold in the rhubarb and spread the batter into the prepared pan. Sprinkle on the topping.

Bake the cake for 35 to 40 minutes, until the center springs back when gently pressed. Let cool on a wire rack for 10 minutes before cutting into 12 rectangles.

CHAPTER SEVEN

SEEDS AND PODS

From fresh *haricots verts* and baby wax beans in the early summer, to fava beans, corn, edamame, and peas midseason, to vine-dried heritage beans at Thanksgiving, CSAs enjoy some member of this vegetable group almost every week.

Members of the Leguminosae, or pulse, family, fresh beans, shell beans, dried beans, corn, okra, and peas are the seeds of their plants and in some cases the edible containers that hold them. Because of their reproductive function, they are one of the most nutritious parts of the plant. And because of the various stages at which they may be used, they bring great variety to the vegetable menu.

Beans are an important part of the heritage of people from all corners of the earth. Simultaneously, different beans were being nurtured and enjoyed in Asia, the Mediterranean, and the Western Hemisphere. Asian cultures perfected the soybean as well as the adzuki and the mung bean. Southern Europe and northern Africa cultivated garbanzo and fava beans, and haricots (from the Aztec "*ayacotl*") and lima beans flourished in North and South America. Centuries of trading between Asia and Europe intensified as ships ventured westward in the fifteenth and sixteenth centuries, and all three bean cultures merged in the stew pots and salad bowls of the world. While Eastern and Mediterranean beans are usually just enjoyed fresh from the pod or dried, many Western beans may be eaten along with the pod when both are immature. This range of possibilities makes it possible to feed your family from the bean patch throughout the growing season and to store a supply of dried beans for later use. CSA members usually find fresh green and wax beans;

mature beans of all kinds to be removed from the shell and cooked fresh; and, at the end of the season, dried beans in their shares.

Corn is central in the food history of North and South America. This interesting seed has been interacting with humans for so long that it cannot reproduce without the help of someone to remove the husks and separate the grains for planting. This versatile vegetable can be eaten in stir-fried dishes when very immature, eaten on or off the cob when full and sweet, and boiled or ground to make meal or flour when mature and dried. The husks can be used for cooking wrappers, the fresh cobs can be simmered to make a wonderful vegetable stock, and the dried cobs can serve as fuel for a cooking fire. Our CSA shares usually have three or four weeks of fresh sweet corn in the middle of the summer.

Peas probably originated in western Asia but were a part of the Mediterranean diet by classical times and were recorded in both Greek and Roman writings. These days, it is common for U.S. farmers to grow three types of peas: the regular garden pea, which is shelled before eating, as well as snow peas and sugar snap peas, which are eaten with the pod. CSA members often get all three in their shares at different times during the season. Garden peas can be allowed to mature and dry on the vine just as beans do for long-term storage.

Okra is a member of the mallow family native to Africa. Brought to colonial America early in the seventeenth century, it is especially traditional in the South. It is succulent and sweet when small but gets woody as it matures.

In the Field

Legumes are fairly easy to grow and don't need much special care. As a group, they add nitrogen to the soil during the growth process, so are perfect for organic farming. Once called string beans, green and wax beans have practically no strings these days. While there is some interest in reviving heritage beans, most of the work has been done with varieties that will be used as shell beans or dried beans, perhaps because no one wants the strings back. It is best to harvest beans as needed by pinching off the stem about ¼ inch above the end of the bean.

If beans are not picked frequently, they become tough and tasteless (and eventually stop producing completely). Corn is a high-maintenance crop but well worth the extra work. It needs fertilization at several points in its development (Native Americans used to plant a fish with each sprinkling of corn seeds).

Corn won't tolerate any frost, so planting it early is risky. Insects love it as much as we do, so organic farmers have to watch it carefully and treat it quickly with organic controls. And organic eaters need to remember that a few chewed-on kernels don't ruin the whole ear—just cut away those parts. New varieties, such as 'Super Sweet,' have been developed to have more sweetness and to resist the conversion of sugar to starch, giving it a longer shelf life.

Okra grows easily in most parts of North America. It is essential to keep an eye on the pods when they first start to arrive in midsummer and harvest them when they are small. They grow from small and succulent to large and useless in the blink of an eye.

Shell peas, sugar snap peas, and snow peas are happier when the weather is cool, so it is no puzzle why they are considered a springtime treat. By midsummer, they are past their prime. Peas also fix nitrogen so require less tending than some other crops. In a home garden, they make a beautiful fence cover with their pretty flowers, and it is much easier to keep an eye on them and harvest them when the peas are of medium size and the pods are still a fresh green.

Selecting the Best

The rules are pretty much the same for selecting fresh beans, peas, and okra. It is important to find them just mature enough to have some seed development, yet young enough to be tender and sweet. Green beans, snow peas, and sugar snap peas are delicious when quite immature. Okra reaches perfection between 2 and 3 inches in length. If they are even a little larger and the pod feels woody when cut or the seeds are dark rather than caramel colored, they are not worth cooking. Garden peas or shell peas should look full but not split or dried out. All should have no dark spots or signs of dryness or mold.

Corn is at its prime when the silk has just started to turn brown. The husks should look fresh and green with no holes or signs of infestation, and the stem end should be green and look freshly broken. Since CSA corn is organic, it is hard not to share some with smaller creatures, but if all the ears have some signs of gnawing, select only those that have no holes in the body of the corn, because the tips can easily be broken off and discarded.

After You Pick Up or Buy

In their fresh state, all the seeds and pods should be used as soon after you get them as possible. Fresh beans, snow peas, sugar snap peas, and okra are quite perishable but can be wrapped tightly and stored overnight in the refrigerator. They should not be washed until you are ready to cook them. Shell beans should be refrigerated in their shells and shelled just before cooking. However, shell peas and corn are really best if cooked immediately after they are harvested. The old adage of starting the water to boil before you go to the field to pick the corn holds true for shell peas as well. Both are high in sugars that turn to starch after harvest. Unfortunately, few of us have the luxury of a cornfield outside our door. But now, fortunately for corn lovers, the newer varieties retain their sweetness much longer. If corn is not going to be cooked right after picking, it should be refrigerated in the husks and husked just before cooking.

Preparing Uncooked

Just before serving, rinse, drain, and remove the stem ends from fresh beans, snow peas, and sugar snap peas. Pull off the strings along the edges of snow peas and sugar snap peas. The pointed ends of fresh beans do not have to be removed unless you want to. As a matter of fact, they look very pretty with the tips on. Any of these may be added to salads, used as crudités or with dips, or packed as lunch-box snacks. To serve corn raw, remove the husks and cut the kernels from the cobs. Toss the corn with other chopped raw vegetables for salads, relishes, or salsas. Okra is not served raw.

Preparing Cooked

BLANCHING is all the cooking fresh green or wax beans, snow peas, sugar snap peas, okra, and corn really need. You want to expose them to the boiling water just long enough to heat them, set their color, and mellow the raw flavor. Two to 4 minutes will do it and you couldn't call that boiling.

To Soak or Not to Soak?

Most dried beans will profit from being soaked before cooking. It helps them to absorb moisture uniformly and cook with less incidence of splitting. Black-eyed peas and lentils are the exception and don't need to be soaked unless they have been stored for a long time. As beans are stored, they get drier and drier, and if they are stored in a warm place, they get even drier. This makes it difficult to tell how long they will need to be soaked and cooked in order to become tender. Beans should be sorted and rinsed before soaking. The easiest way to soak beans is to cover them with water in a bowl, cover the bowl with plastic wrap, and refrigerate them overnight. The fastest way to soak beans is to bring them to a boil in water to cover. Cover the saucepan and set it off the heat for 1 hour. After soaking, discard the water, rinse the beans again, and they are ready to cook. If you don't have time to soak them, bring them to a boil in a very large pot of water; cover it and simmer until they are tender, which may be as short as 1 hour or as long as 2.

BOILING is the best choice for shell peas, shell beans, and dried beans. These vary in dryness depending upon their maturity or, in the case of dried beans, upon storage conditions. Fresh shell peas and shell beans should be ready to serve in 10 to 15 minutes. For more on cooking dried beans, see To Soak or Not to Soak? above.

DEEP-FRYING adds crunch to okra. Dip whole small pods or ½-inch pieces in batter or cornmeal and fry quickly until crisp and brown.

GRILLING really brings out the flavor of corn on the cob. Some people say corn is more flavorful if it's cooked in its husk. On the other hand, it takes several minutes more to cook and it's much harder to take off the husk when it's hot. Either way, rinse the corn and remove the silk before grilling for about 3 minutes without the husk or 5 with it, turning occasionally.

MICROWAVING is an easy way to cook one ear of corn for a snack. Remove the husk and silk, rinse and place on a microwavable saucer or a piece of wax

Edamame

Edible soybeans are related to, and have the same high nutritional values and protein levels as, regular soybeans, but they're much easier to cook and are eaten in the fresh shell stage rather than dried, making them much more digestible. According to the Johnny's Selected Seeds catalog, they not only are better adapted to northern growing conditions than limas (to which they taste similar) but also have more protein and better yields.

To prepare edamame, strip the pods from the branches, but don't shell them. Rinse them, then steam or boil them in salted water for about 5 minutes. Rinse with cold water to cool the pods, then shell by popping the beans out of the pods. Don't overcook; they're better when they are a little crisp. Dress them with unsalted butter or any sauce, add them to a stir-fry, or just serve them in their pods and pop out to eat, like peanuts. When we asked the children of our CSA which vegetable they liked best, edamame easily won, probably because it is so much fun to eat. If you have more than you can use in several days, they freeze very well.

paper, and microwave on high power for 3 minutes. Turn over and microwave on high for 2 minutes more.

STEAMING will cook green or wax beans and corn to perfection. The beans will take 3 to 5 minutes, depending upon their size and how many you are cooking, and the corn will take about 7 minutes.

STIR-FRYING can make a meal of green or wax beans, snow peas or sugar snap peas, blanched shell peas or shell beans, okra, and corn that has been taken off the cob. Add any of these for the last 5 minutes of the cooking time for the dish.

Preserving

Although green and wax beans may be canned, freezing is certainly the best choice for preserving any of the seeds and pods. All should be blanched before freezing. Pack them in glass or plastic freezer containers and store them at 0°F for up to a year. Dried beans, of course, may be kept in a tight container at room temperature. It is best to keep them in a cool, dry place because heat causes them to dry out and to take an excessive time to reconstitute, while humidity can cause spoilage.

Seed and Pod Nutrition

Fresh green beans are high in fiber, potassium, and vitamins A and C. Wax beans have similar nutrient content, except they do not have the vitamin A. Dried beans are rich in carbohydrates, contain a decent supply of incomplete protein, and are rich in iron, phosphorus, and potassium. Corn contains reasonable amounts of vitamins A, B, and C, potassium, and fiber. And corn kernels contain an incomplete protein; combine corn with legumes (like soybeans) or a little animal protein (like eggs or cheese), and the protein is complete. Peas are high in carbohydrates, vitamins A and C, thiamin, riboflavin, niacin, phosphorus, iron, and potassium. Not to be left out, okra provides enough vitamin C, iron, and calcium to be recognized.

Sprouts

Originally considered an Asian ingredient, bean sprouts have gone mainstream and regularly appear in salads, casseroles, and stir-fries these days. To make them at home, start with edible, organic beans, never with beans intended for planting. You may be able to find a bean sprout kit at a natural foods store. Pick over and rinse the beans. Cover the beans with water in a medium bowl and set aside, covered, in a cool place to soak overnight. Next day, drain well; cover the bowl with cheesecloth and tie securely in place. Let stand at room temperature in a dark place for 3 to 4 days, until the sprouts are the desired length, rinsing and draining once a day. (You can do this through the cheesecloth.)

SKAGIT LEEK, POTATO, AND PEA SOUP

MAKES 8 SERVINGS

Suzanne Butler, manager of the Skagit Valley Farmers' Market in northwest Washington State, contributed this recipe, which she developed to include the best of the springtime produce in her market. She is a member of Chefs Collaborative and has been Graham Kerr's cooking assistant for the past ten years. Her passion for fresh local food has led her to become active in the struggle to save farmlands in her county, and this includes managing the market.

4 cups sliced leeks, cleaned, white parts
   with a little of the light green only
4 cups chopped peeled russet potatoes
1/2 teaspoon salt
2 cups thawed frozen green peas
1 cup half-and-half or evaporated
   2% milk, plus more as needed
1 tablespoon lemon juice

1/4 teaspoon freshly milled white
   pepper
2 cups 1/2-inch cubes scrubbed red
   potatoes
1 cup frozen petits pois
1/4 cup finely chopped fresh parsley
1/4 cup finely chopped fresh chives
Chive flowers for garnish (optional)

Combine 7 cups water with the leeks, russet potatoes, and salt in a large pan. Bring to a boil, cover partially, and simmer for 25 minutes, or until the potatoes are very tender. Set aside until cool enough to work with.

Puree the mixture in a food processor with the thawed green peas until smooth. Push through a sieve back into the soup kettle. Stir in the half-and-half, lemon juice, and white pepper. Bring just to a boil.

Meanwhile, steam the red potatoes for about 10 minutes, or until barely tender. Add to the soup with the frozen petits pois and stir until heated through, 1 or 2 minutes. Thin with a little more half-and-half and add salt, if necessary. Serve garnished with a mix of the parsley and chives. Chives flowers will add a nice touch.

This recipe is from New York's Canticle Farm, sponsored by the Franciscan Sisters of Allegany, a religious order whose mission is "to reverence, protect, and honor the sacredness of God's creation." Their CSA is committed to connecting all peoples and to practicing earth-friendly habits.

CORN CHOWDER

MAKES 4 SERVINGS

1 tablespoon unsalted butter
1 cup chopped green and red bell
   pepper
1 cup sliced celery
1 cup chopped onions
2 potatoes, peeled and diced
Chopped fresh basil and parsley

2 bay leaves
Salt and freshly milled black pepper
1 teaspoon paprika, cayenne, or a
   Louisiana-style spice blend
2 cups fresh or frozen corn kernels
2 cups milk
2 cups heavy cream

Melt the butter over medium heat in a medium Dutch oven. Add the bell pepper, celery, and onions; sauté until soft, about 5 minutes.

Add the potatoes and 3 cups hot water. Stir in basil and parsley to taste, the bay leaves, salt and pepper to taste, and the paprika. Cook, covered, until the potatoes are crisp-tender.

Puree half of the corn and add it to the vegetables. Add the rest of the corn along with the milk and the cream. Heat just to a boil; remove bay leaves, garnish with additional chopped basil and parsley, and serve.

CHEDDAR CORN PUDDING

MAKES 8 SIDE-DISH SERVINGS
OR 4 MAIN-DISH SERVINGS

Kevin von Klause, executive chef/partner at the White Dog Café in Philadelphia, told us that "the privilege of buying directly from farmers is one that we never take for granted. We are delighted to prepare for our guests the farm-fresh products we receive each week from almost thirty local producers. Their passion for food is as evident as any chef's that I have ever known. The farmers determine our menu offerings with their weekly harvest, and they stir our creative juices with the abundance of their toils." He added that this recipe is an old favorite in the White Dog kitchen and that they serve it with roasted chicken for dinner, with sliced country ham for brunch, and with a green salad and sliced tomatoes for a quick and satisfying lunch.

8 tablespoons (1 stick) unsalted butter
2 cups finely chopped onions
3 tablespoons chopped fresh thyme,
    or 1½ tablespoons dried
½ cup all-purpose flour
2 cups heavy cream

8 cups fresh corn kernels
6 large eggs
2 cups grated Cheddar cheese
2 teaspoons salt
1 teaspoon freshly milled black pepper

Preheat the oven to 350°F. Lightly butter or coat with vegetable spray a 13-by 9-inch baking dish.

Melt the butter in a large, heavy skillet over medium heat. Add the onions and thyme and sauté until the onions are very soft, about 6 minutes. Stir in the flour until completely incorporated. Transfer to a medium mixing bowl; stir in 1 cup of the cream and let the mixture cool to lukewarm.

Combine 4 cups of the corn kernels with the eggs and the remaining 1 cup cream in the bowl of a food processor. Process until just smooth. Add to the onion mixture along with the remaining 4 cups corn kernels and the Cheddar cheese, salt, and pepper. Mix well. Pour the corn mixture into the buttered baking dish. Bake for 30 minutes, or until a knife inserted in the center comes out clean. Serve warm.

Patricia Janof of the Carnegie Hill/Yorkville CSA in Manhattan likes to make this when she gets her share of dried 'Jacob's Cattle' beans at the end of the season. She says, "This recipe is very adaptable. A thinner broth and smaller vegetables lends itself to soup. You can add cooked cubed chicken or other meat near the end of the cooking time, if you wish."

END-OF-SUMMER STEW

MAKES 6 SERVINGS

4 to 5 garlic cloves
1 tablespoon olive oil
1 large onion, coarsely chopped
1 tablespoon ground cumin
1 (28-ounce) can tomatoes, whole or chopped, with juice (if whole, cut into pieces)
2 to 3 cups cubed, scrubbed red potatoes
2 large carrots, coarsely chopped

1 cup sliced fresh green beans
1 cup fresh corn kernels
1 (15-ounce) can black-eyed peas or 2 cups cooked dried beans, drained
2 tablespoons chopped fresh parsley
2 tablespoons chopped fresh basil, or 2 teaspoons dried (optional)
1 tablespoon chopped fresh oregano, or 1 teaspoon dried (optional)
Salt and freshly milled black pepper

Finely chop the garlic; set aside for 15 minutes. Heat the oil in a large pot; add the onion and garlic. Sauté them until just golden, about 4 minutes. Add the cumin and cook, stirring, for about 2 minutes.

Add the tomatoes, potatoes, and carrots to the pot; cook for 15 minutes. Add the green beans, corn, and black-eyed peas; cook for 10 minutes. Stir in the parsley, basil and oregano, if using, and salt and pepper to taste. Cook for 5 minutes more, or until all the vegetables are tender.

Meet the Farmer

Angelic Organics, Caledonia, Illinois

John Peterson and his two sisters grew up on their parents' dairy farm in Caledonia, Illinois, some one hundred miles northwest of Chicago in the rolling hills along the Illinois-Wisconsin border. John, who is also a writer, didn't always plan to be a farmer.

He was nineteen and attending nearby Beloit College when his father became ill. Though John had always helped around the farm, it was only then that he really stepped up to the plate. So, at an age when many young men and women clash with their parents and leave the family homestead, John got a chance to manage the farm and try out some of his own ideas. Many of them didn't work, but he was hooked on farming anyway.

"If I'm on a tractor, I'm happy," says John, who ultimately bought the farm from his mother. "I like bins and boxes overflowing with produce and fields packed with crops. Maybe it flies in the face of 'small is beautiful,' but I just happen to love and revel in abundance."

John tried a number of scenarios at the farm before settling on the CSA concept in 1992. Shortly after his father died, John sold off the cows and began raising corn and beans. He then tried raising hogs, mistakenly thinking that pigs would be more lucrative than plants. They weren't. John almost lost the farm when commodity prices collapsed in the early 1980s. He had to auction off equipment and most of the land except for the farmstead. John wrote a play about the losses and toured the state with it.

Finally, he decided to try an organic vegetable farm, which later evolved according to the bio-dynamic nonchemical farming philosophy developed by Rudolph Steiner. After some Chicagoans approached him about starting a CSA (and he overcame some misgivings about the idea of non-farmers telling him how to farm), he started a pilot program with thirty shareholders. John has been operating the now eighty-five-acre farm as a CSA ever since. It is now one of the country's largest CSAs, as it serves some one thousand shareholders.

John, who often writes essays on farming for the CSA newsletter, is also working on compiling his farming stories into a book that may soon be available on the farm's website (*www.angelic-organics.com*) along with a cookbook that will ultimately replace the weekly newsletter recipes.

John loves to grow sweet corn and has always been fascinated with the great green swaths of corn that blanket the Midwest. There's something about the stalks' uprightness swaying in the wind that is mesmerizing and almost oceanlike. And the process of picking corn by snapping it decisively off the stalk is very satisfying, he says. "So many people talk about how horrible it is to drive across the Midwest because all there is are cornfields," John says, "but I love it. It's amazing."

Diane Franklin of Rocky Gardens CSA in Davisburg, Michigan, says, "Every summer when the beans start to come in, my family gets excited for this dinner. And anyone who has ever made it reports back to me how much the family enjoyed it." She says that she grows a firm Spanish-type green bean that needs a few more minutes of cooking than the potatoes, but that not all types of beans will need this.

GREEN BEANS, POTATOES, AND SAUSAGE

MAKES 4 SERVINGS

1 pound smoked sausage or lite smoked sausage
1 pound fresh green beans, trimmed and cut in half
1/2 teaspoon garlic salt
1/2 teaspoon Maggie's seasoning or soy sauce
12 ounces small red potatoes, scrubbed and quartered

Cut the sausage diagonally into 1/2-inch slices. Put the sausage and beans into a large pot with water to cover. Add the garlic salt and Maggie's seasoning. Bring the water to a boil, add the potatoes, and simmer, stirring occasionally, for 15 to 20 minutes. Depending on the type of green beans you use, the length of time you cook the potatoes and beans together could be different. You want both the beans and the potatoes to be tender but not mushy. Serve this right from the pot with bread or rolls and some sliced fresh tomatoes.

CATFISH IN CORN HUSKS WITH SWEET BODACIOUS CORN RELISH AND CHILI BUTTER

MAKES 12 SERVINGS

Sylvia Oliveira, executive chef of Bon Appétit at Hewlett-Packard in Boise, Idaho, sent us this recipe. She makes it with Hagerman farm-raised catfish. When we asked her about her support of sustainable agriculture and her work as a chef, she told us, "I hope to be a contributing part of the cycle, much like my ancestors, so that small farmers and producers may survive long into the future."

1 (1-pound) package dry corn husks
½ pound (2 sticks) unsalted butter, softened
3 tablespoons ancho chili powder
3 garlic cloves, finely chopped
6 ears 'Sweet Bodacious' or other sweet corn
1 red bell pepper, chopped
1 medium red onion, chopped
4 jalapeño peppers, seeded and chopped
2 tablespoons chopped fresh cilantro
2 tablespoons chopped pink pickled sushi ginger
Salt and freshly milled black pepper
12 (6-ounce) catfish fillets

The day before serving, rinse the corn husks and cover them with boiling water in a large bowl. Set aside to cool to room temperature, then cover and refrigerate overnight. Beat the butter in a medium bowl with an electric mixer until fluffy. Add the chili powder and garlic; beat until combined. Transfer the mixture to a piece of parchment or wax paper and shape into a log 2½ inches in diameter. Wrap the parchment around the butter and roll to smooth the sides. Wrap tightly in plastic wrap and freeze.

About an hour before serving, husk and clean the corn. Slice the kernels from the cobs and place in a medium bowl with the bell pepper, onion, jalapeño peppers, cilantro, ginger, and salt and pepper to taste. Set aside. Rinse and drain the soaked husks; set aside 24 large husks (about 6 inches in length) and tear the smaller husks with the grain to make 24 strips (about ¼ inch wide) for ties. Slice the frozen chili butter into 24 pieces.

To assemble, place two 6-inch corn husks on a work surface with the wide ends overlapping in the center to make a 10-inch wrapper. Place a fillet, skin side down, on the husks and season with salt and pepper. Top it with 3 tablespoons of the corn mixture and 2 chili butter slices. Roll the fish in the corn husk to make a log about 10 inches long. Tie the ends closed at the place where the fillet ends. Steam the packets for 12 to 15 minutes, until they feel firm; serve immediately.

Meet the Farmers

Bluebird Hills Farm, Springfield, Ohio

Tim and Laurel Shouvlin both grew up living next door to farms. But, though Laurel acknowledges that their last name is perfect for their current occupation, neither went right into farming. In their former lives, Tim was an attorney and Laurel was formally trained as a physician's assistant. The land beckoned them back in 1992, when the couple bought five hundred acres in southwestern Ohio on the edge of the corn belt. They are now full-time farmers. They raise alpaca and run a CSA farm with nearly two hundred shareholders.

Bluebird Hills Farm is a mix of hilly pastures, flat tillable land, and wooded acreage. The Shouvlins cultivate only about thirty of the acres simultaneously. The farm is dotted with bluebird boxes that the Shouvlins provide for nesting. The once-common birds have become a rare sight because their habitat has been diminished by development.

Why did Tim and Laurel decide to start a CSA? Like many farmers, they grew tired of the unpredictability of farmers' markets. "That was pretty tough," Laurel says. "If there was an Ohio State football game, nobody showed up. This was a much more guaranteed approach." That's not to say that CSAs are for the fainthearted, or for those who have never grown vegetables before. In fact, Laurel was at first very leery of being on the hook to people who paid on the barrel (and ahead of time) for their vegetables. "I felt awkward being indebted," she recalls. But so far, so good. Since the CSA got under way with their first season in 2000, Laurel and her husband have been able to deliver on their promise of weekly certified organic produce.

"It's not uncommon for people to say, 'I haven't tasted a tomato like this since my grandmother grew it in her backyard," Laurel says. What makes Bluebird's tomatoes so sweet? Laurel swears by cover-cropping and composting, organic farming practices that put necessary micronutrients back into the soil. "You just don't get that when you pop open a bag of fertilizer." In addition, the Shouvlins don't need to plant varieties that will ship well. They choose varieties that will taste great. Brandywines are their favorite.

SALADE NIÇOISE WITH GRILLED AHI TUNA

MAKES 4 SERVINGS

Ross Browne, executive chef of Absinthe Brasserie and Bar in San Francisco, brings classic flavor to his salade Niçoise with fresh ahi tuna, salt-roasted potatoes, oil-cured olives, and locally grown organic *haricots verts,* wax beans, and heirloom tomatoes. He recommends rinsing the olives and capers ahead of time to reduce their saltiness and then storing them in a peppery extra-virgin olive oil.

12 fingerling or baby new potatoes, scrubbed
4 garlic cloves, unpeeled
4 fresh thyme sprigs
1 tablespoon unsalted butter
Salt and freshly milled black pepper
8 ounces fresh green beans, preferably haricots verts, trimmed
8 ounces fresh yellow beans, trimmed
1 to 1¼ pounds ahi tuna, cut into 4 equal pieces
½ teaspoon crushed coriander seeds

Peppery extra-virgin olive oil
1 large yellow tomato, cut into 12 wedges
20 Niçoise olives, rinsed and pitted
4 anchovy fillets, sliced lengthwise into strips (optional)
2 tablespoons capers, rinsed
12 fresh tarragon leaves
½ teaspoon chopped fresh chervil
Red wine vinegar
2 large red tomatoes, cut into 12 slices
1 cup mixed miniature greens

Preheat the oven to 425°F. Place the potatoes, garlic, thyme, and butter on a sheet of parchment paper or aluminum foil. Sprinkle with ½ teaspoon salt and ¼ teaspoon pepper. Wrap the parchment tightly around the potatoes; place on a rimmed baking sheet and roast for 25 to 30 minutes. Open the packet and discard the garlic and thyme; set the potatoes aside to cool slightly.

Meanwhile, bring 3 inches of salted water to a boil in each of 2 medium saucepans. Add the green beans to one and the yellow beans to the other; return to a boil. Boil the beans for 30 seconds; drain and set aside to cool slightly. If the beans are large, cut them in half.

Rub the tuna with the coriander seeds and ¼ teaspoon black pepper. Heat 1 tablespoon olive oil in a large, heavy skillet over medium heat. Add the tuna and sear on both sides. Remove to a platter, or cook longer, if desired, and then remove and set aside to come to room temperature.

Combine the potatoes, green and yellow beans, yellow tomato wedges, olives, anchovies, if using, capers, tarragon, and chervil in a large bowl. Add oil, vinegar, salt, and pepper to taste; toss gently to combine.

To serve, on each of 4 large chilled plates, arrange 3 red tomato slices; season with oil, vinegar, salt, and pepper to taste. Top with the bean mixture and tuna. Sprinkle the miniature greens over the top and serve.

At Common Ground Farm in Spring Mills, Pennsylvania, Leslie Zuck and her family grow nutritious organic produce for the local community. They are dedicated to the land, nurturing the soil and acting as responsible stewards in their relationship with the earth and what it can provide. Common Ground also provides the opportunity for volunteer apprentices to experience daily life on a certified organic farm. By assisting the organic farmer, the apprentice learns what it takes to create a successful organic farming system.

MEDITERRANEAN BEANS AND TOMATOES

MAKES 6 SERVINGS

1 tablespoon olive oil
1 small onion, thinly sliced
2 garlic cloves, finely chopped
3 large tomatoes, seeded and chopped
1 tablespoon chopped fresh basil, oregano, or parsley

Salt and freshly milled black pepper
1 1/2 pounds fresh green, wax, or purple beans, trimmed
1/2 pound feta cheese, crumbled
1/4 pound green or black olives, halved or sliced

Heat the oil in a large saucepan over medium heat. Add the onion and sauté until translucent, about 4 minutes. Add the garlic; cook 1 minute more.

Stir in the tomatoes, basil, and salt and pepper to taste. Cook until the tomatoes are wilted, 4 to 5 minutes. Stir in the beans and cook until they are heated through and just crisp-tender, 3 to 5 minutes more. Top with feta cheese and olives; toss quickly. Serve immediately.

ASIAN-INDIAN OKRA AND TOMATOES

MAKES 4 SERVINGS

Mountain Harvest Organics is nestled in a valley shadowed by beautiful Bluff Mountain, over which the Appalachian Trail passes. The farm belongs to the Appalachian Sustainable Agriculture Project (ASAP), which is a western North Carolina community-based collaborative focused on sustaining farms and rural communities through an integrated-action program. This northern Indian recipe is a favorite of farmers Julie Mansfield and Carl Evans, who frequently cook Asian-Indian dishes because they love their wonderful combination of spices. They told us, "Cooking okra with tomatoes, tamarind, lemon juice, or dry mango powder eliminates the slimy effect okra often has when cooked."

¾ teaspoon ground cumin
¼ teaspoon ground coriander
⅛ teaspoon cayenne
⅛ teaspoon ground fennel
⅛ teaspoon ground turmeric
3 tablespoons light vegetable oil
4 ounces okra, rinsed, drained, and trimmed, left whole if small or cut into bite-sized pieces

¾ cup finely chopped onions
2 garlic cloves, finely chopped
1 tablespoon finely chopped peeled fresh ginger
¾ cup finely chopped tomatoes
Salt
1 tablespoon chopped fresh cilantro

Measure the cumin, coriander, cayenne, fennel, and turmeric into a small bowl. Heat 1 tablespoon of the oil in a large, heavy skillet over medium-high heat. When the oil is very hot, add the okra in a single layer and fry without stirring for 1 minute. Continue cooking for 3 to 4 minutes more, tossing and turning the okra until it is lightly browned. Remove the okra from the pan and set aside.

Add the remaining 2 tablespoons oil to the same pan along with the onions. Cook the onions, stirring occasionally, until light golden, about 5 minutes. Add the garlic and ginger and cook, stirring constantly, until the mixture caramelizes, 8 to 10 minutes. Add the spices; stir for a few seconds and then add the tomatoes and ¼ cup water.

Reduce the heat to medium and cook, stirring, for 3 minutes, or until the mixture thickens. Add the fried okra and salt to taste. Return to a boil and cook, covered, over low heat, until the okra is cooked and the sauce thickens, about 20 minutes. Stir in 1½ teaspoons of the cilantro, and garnish with the remaining 1½ teaspoons.

This recipe was contributed by Waldy Malouf, chef/owner of Beacon Restaurant in Manhattan. He told us, "Here, I grill or roast shucked ears so the kernels develop a concentrated toasted-corn flavor and take on some char. The kernels are then sliced from the cobs and served with fresh shell beans, basil-flecked tomatoes, and savory red onions and scallions."

SMOKY CORN SUCCOTASH

MAKES 6 SERVINGS

2 cups fresh shelled cranberry beans
   (from 1½ pounds)
6 ears fresh corn, husks removed
3 medium tomatoes
2 tablespoons extra-virgin olive oil
1 tablespoon chopped fresh basil

Coarse sea salt or kosher salt and
   freshly milled black pepper
2 cups diced red onions
¾ cup chopped green onions
4 tablespoons (½ stick) unsalted
   butter

Place the beans in a large pot. Add enough water to cover them by 1 inch and bring to a boil. Reduce the heat, partially cover the pot, and simmer for about 1 hour. The beans should be soft and creamy but still separate and intact. Watch carefully to make sure that they do not burn, adding more water, if necessary, as the beans cook. There should be at least 1 cup of liquid remaining in the pot when the beans are cooked. The beans can be made a few hours in advance and reheated gently in their liquid.

Preheat the grill. Place the ears on the grill and cook, turning occasionally, until they just start to turn brown around the edges, about 10 minutes.

Let the corn cool. Holding the corn in a large bowl, run a sharp knife along the cobs to cut away all the kernels, then run the back of the knife along the cobs to scrape the liquid into the bowl. Set aside.

In a bowl, mix together the tomatoes, olive oil, basil, and salt and pepper to taste. Place the diced onions and chopped green onions in separate serving bowls.

When ready to serve, put the beans, 1 cup of the reserved cooking liquid, and 2 tablespoons of the butter in a small saucepan. Cook over medium heat until the butter melts. Season to taste with salt and pepper. Transfer the beans to a serving bowl. Place the corn, their juice, and the remaining 2 tablespoons butter in a small saucepan and heat until the butter melts and the corn is heated through. Season with salt and pepper to taste. Transfer to a serving bowl.

Serve the bowls of vegetables while the beans and corn are still warm. Let people assemble their own plates of succotash to taste.

GRILLED CORN ON THE COB WITH LIME RUB

MAKES 4 SERVINGS

Ronna N. Welsh, sous-chef at Danal Restaurant in Manhattan, gave us this spicy recipe. When we asked her about the interesting mix of spices, she told us, "This is the only time I use garlic powder when I cook. I find that it gives the spice mix enough of an earthy undertone without undoing the corn's sweetness and the lime's tang. You can also do this recipe directly over the flames of a gas stove, provided you have enough burners to go around."

4 ears fresh corn, stems attached, husks removed
2 tablespoons ground toasted cumin seeds
2 tablespoons garlic powder
2 tablespoons hot paprika or 1 ½ tablespoons paprika and ½ tablespoon ground red pepper
2 tablespoons salt
2 limes, cut into 8 wedges

Preheat a charcoal grill. Rinse and dry the corn. Arrange the corn on the grill over hot coals and cook, turning occasionally by their stems, until charred all around, 4 to 6 minutes.

Meanwhile, combine the cumin, garlic powder, paprika, and salt in a small bowl. Immediately as the corn comes off the grill, dip a wedge of lime or two into the spice mixture and squeeze and rub it all over the surface of the corn. Eat while hot.

Chef Christopher Hastings of the Hot and Hot Fish Club in Birmingham, Alabama, serves this cornmeal-coated fried okra as a topping on his heritage tomato salad along with crumbled bacon and vinaigrette-dressed butter beans and corn. A creamy chive dressing is drizzled over all the ingredients. When we asked Chef Hastings about the ingredients around which he designs the restaurant's menu, he told us, "As a chef, I have spent my entire career searching the country for the highest-quality, often local, wild or organic meat, fish, and produce to express our commitment to clean, honest, seasonal cooking."

FRIED OKRA

MAKES 6 SERVINGS ON A TOMATO SALAD OR 4 SIDE-DISH SERVINGS

30 small okra, rinsed and drained
1/4 cup buttermilk
1/4 cup corn flour
1/4 cup cornmeal
1/4 cup all-purpose flour

1/8 to 1/4 teaspoon salt
1/8 teaspoon freshly milled black pepper
4 cups vegetable oil

Trim off the stems of the okra leaving the caps intact. Toss the okra with the buttermilk in a small bowl. Combine the corn flour, cornmeal, all-purpose flour, salt, and pepper in a medium bowl.

Heat the vegetable oil to 350°F in a small saucepan. Drain the okra and toss in the corn flour mixture. Fry in several batches until golden brown, about 3 minutes; drain on paper towels. Taste and add more salt and pepper, if desired, and serve on a tomato salad or as a side dish.

How to Boil Corn on the Cob

Boiled corn on the cob is one of America's favorite summertime treats. And the recipe elicits sur-prisingly strong feelings for such a short list of ingredients. If you ask home cooks, they will all pretty much tell you that you need to rush the corn from the field to the boiling water; but then the dif-ferences begin. Cooking times vary from as long as an hour to as short as 30 seconds. Some people like to add nothing to the water but the corn, while others insist on salt, pepper, sugar, or all three. We're willing to bet that you have a special way that pleases you, so don't change a thing, but if you don't have a special way, why don't you try this? Plunge the freshly husked corn into a large pot of rapidly boiling salted water. Turn off the heat immediately and let the corn stand for 3 minutes. Re-move it immediately and serve it with lots of butter and some kosher salt on the side.

CHAPTER EIGHT

FRUITS OF THE VEGETABLE WORLD

They're the stars of the vegetable world, and when they're around, they take center stage. Be honest, how many people wait for the first head of cabbage with the same anticipation as they do the first tomato of the season? Which vegetables do we turn to when we want to add substance and color to a meal? Not kale or celery, but peppers, eggplant, zucchini. And do you think it's an accident that Cinderella's fairy godmother passed over rutabagas and onions and chose a plump orange pumpkin to become a golden carriage?

Fruits contain the future, the seeds of the next generation. Botanically, a fruit is the plant's ovary, so tomatoes, eggplant, peppers, cucumbers, and squash are fruits even though they don't grow on trees. The foods we commonly call fruits—the ones that do grow on trees—are often sweeter, but fresh vegetable fruits also have a high sugar content and are juicy and delicious enough to be used in cakes, breads, and desserts.

Vegetable fruits fall into two families: cucurbits (cucumbers and squash, along with melons, which you'll find in chapter 11) and nightshades (tomatoes, eggplant, peppers). Each has its own attributes.

THE CUCURBITS

Most of the members of this family come from the tropics and subtropics. Cucumbers originated in India and other warm regions of Asia and were grown as far back as three thousand years ago. The adjective that's associated with them is "cool," and if you've ever placed cucumber slices over your eyes or rubbed one over your skin, you'll know how appropriate this connection is (you'll also have benefited from cucumber's substantial vitamin E, which is an excellent skin conditioner). Squash are South American natives; they were unknown in the rest of the world before Columbus's voyages but were added to the cuisines of Europe and Asia not long after they were introduced. By the eighteenth century, they were worldwide staples. Thin-skinned summer squash and hard-shelled winter squash are actually the same vegetable at different stages of development. (Pumpkins are a form of winter squash.) The varieties that we use first are those bred to be cooked briefly (they can even be eaten raw), and we pick them when they're young and juicy (if you leave a summer squash on the vine too long, it will become hard). We allow winter squash varieties to harden on the vine, and their thick shells make it possible for them to be stored for several months. The dense flesh under that shell needs long, slow cooking—roasting winter squash brings out their sweet, nutty flavor best—but they're among the easiest vegetables to use.

In the Field

Cucumbers and squash grow on long vining plants; they're space hogs and each plant needs about fifteen square feet of soil. If the weather agrees with them, they will produce vast quantities of fruit for several weeks, which can sometimes become more of a challenge than a thrill. Before the fruits develop, the vines produce showy yellow flowers; squash blossoms are an edible delicacy (see page 168).

Heat-loving cucumbers stop producing once nights begin to cool. The two main types of cucumber are thin-skinned slicers and thicker-skinned pickling cucumbers. Though we've become used to seeing uniformly sized dark green cukes in the supermarket, CSAs and farm stands often offer a great variety: stubby yellow 'Lemon' or 'Boothbay Blonde' heirlooms, curly Mideastern varieties that grow up to two feet long, and pale green or striped varieties that are nearly seedless.

Summer squash also love hot weather. Once squash fruit appear, they grow amazingly fast—if you don't pick them small, they'll balloon into huge, clublike things that are tasteless and spongy. Squash plants have to be picked frequently because they will shut down production if large, seedy fruit are left on the vine; otherwise, they'll continue to produce new fruit until the first frost. In the past twenty years, zucchini, which are just one type of summer squash, have become supermarket staples. Yellow squash (crookneck and straight types), pale green Mideast types, and flattened pattypans (which are great for stuffing) are prepared in much the same way. Look for dark-and-light-green-striped 'Costata Romanesco,' which has a lower water content than many squash and is better for frying, and creamy-yellow skinned 'Tromboncino,' a superlong, curly squash that has an unusual nutty flavor.

Though winter squash are planted around the same time as summer squash, they're left on the vine to harden for several additional weeks—they need up to 150 days in the field—and will store better if allowed to cure in a dry, shady spot for a few weeks after that. The vines and fruit won't survive frost, though, so they must all be harvested before winter. Though they look very different, most winter squash, from single-serving 'Buttercups' and 'Delicatas' to huge 'Hubbards' and pumpkins, are prepared in the same way; only the length of baking time varies with size. Their flesh ranges from pale orange to bright gold, with some bluish and beige varieties. Some of the tastiest flesh is found in 'Long Island Cheese' pumpkins (a favorite for pies); Delicata (usually about twelve inches long and striped yellow-and-green); and 'Carnival' (a splashy, orange-gold-green acorn type).

Selecting the Best

Cucumbers and summer squash have a high water content and fragile skin. They should be brightly colored, fresh-looking, and firm. Avoid any that look dry at the stem end and have patches of skin missing. Winter squash should have a tough outer shell and feel heavy for their size. Check large squash to see that the area that was resting on the ground has no splits or mold.

After You Pick Up or Buy

Cucumbers and summer squash will last about a week in the crisper drawer of the refrigerator. Store them loose or in open plastic bags. Once they're cut, however, they deteriorate almost immediately, so don't plan to store a started cuke or squash—just eat it. The sweeter varieties of winter squash, like 'Delicata,' 'Buttercup,' and 'Sweet Dumpling,' do not store as well as Hubbards, butternuts, or turbans. They keep better in the refrigerator, so if you have room, place them in the crisper, loose or in open plastic bags, and they'll last for several weeks. Large pumpkins and squash will survive for several weeks even outside the refrigerator—and they are decorative additions to any kitchen counter—but watch them for rot, because when they begin to go, they go quickly.

Preparing Cucumbers

Cucumbers can be sautéed briefly (2 to 3 minutes) in butter if they're salted and drained to remove some of their water first; they can also be steamed for 3 to 4 minutes. But why bother? They're great raw—in salads and as snacks. For a simple, refreshing soup, just throw a few sliced cucumbers (seeds removed or not) into a blender with some vegetable or chicken stock, then stir in plain yogurt or sour cream, mint, salt, and pepper and chill. Cucumber slices and spears are convenient dippers, and hollowed-out cucumber halves or slices are edible holders for shrimp or tuna salads or creamy spreads.

Fresh CSA cucumbers don't have to be peeled; just wash them when you're ready to use them. You can create an interesting effect by scoring unpeeled cucumbers with a knife or fork before slicing. Supermarket cucumbers are often waxed, though, and therefore should be peeled or washed thoroughly before eating.

Preparing Summer Squash

Rinse but don't peel summer squash. Spears and matchsticks make excellent crudités and additions to summer salads. Or cook them in any of the following ways:

MICROWAVING is especially useful when preparing one or two servings. Cut 8 ounces of squash into slices and place into in a microwave-safe dish. Cover, cook on high for about a minute, turn and stir, then cook on high for another minute. Let the squash stand, covered, for a minute before opening.

ROASTING is efficient when you are heating the oven for something else. Slice or quarter large squash; cut small squash in half. Brush with oil; sprinkle with herbs or salt. Place in a 400°F oven for 10 to 15 minutes, until soft.

SAUTÉING adds flavor to the normally mild squash. Slice, dice, quarter, or halve (for small squash) the squash. Heat 2 tablespoons olive oil in a skillet over high heat; if desired, add 2 tablespoons chopped fresh parsley or 2 cloves chopped garlic and sauté briefly. Drop the squash, a handful at a time, and let each batch gain a little color before adding the next batch. The squash will be golden and tender in about 7 minutes. Season with salt and freshly milled black pepper to taste. Serve as is, or over pasta, fish, or rice.

STEAMING preserves the moistness of squash as well as the vitamins. Cut the squash into pieces (matchsticks, rounds, or spears) and place in a steamer basket over boiling water. Cook, covered, until just crisp-tender, 2 to 4 minutes for matchsticks or very young squash, 6 to 8 minutes for halves or larger squash.

Winter squash needs quite a bit of cooking time but very little preparation.

Preparing Winter Squash

BAKING works particularly well for small varieties. Cut the squash lengthwise and scrape out the seeds and stringy portions. You can slice off a small piece at the bottom of each half so that it sits securely. If you have trouble slicing through the squash's hard skin, just puncture it in a few places and put the squash in the oven whole for about 15 minutes. It will then be soft enough to cut easily. Brush the flesh with melted unsalted butter, then drizzle with brown sugar, maple syrup, or honey. Bake for about 30 minutes in a 400°F oven.

BOILING is a quick way to cook winter squash if you cut it into small pieces. Winter squash can be peeled, cut into chunks, and boiled in a big pot of water, but peeling and cutting is not easy. Even if you're boiling, bake for 10 to 15 minutes to soften the skin and the flesh. Save the cooking water (for up to several hours) to cook pasta or rice, which will become infused with the squash's flavor.

MICROWAVING will really reduce squash cooking time. Cut winter squash in half and scrape out the seeds and strings. Wrap each half in microwave-safe plastic wrap and microwave on high for 5 minutes for each 8 ounces of squash.

PUREEING winter squash is the first step for many recipes, including pumpkin pie. To make winter squash puree, cook 1 large or 2 small squash in any of the ways listed here. Then scoop out the meat and put it in a food processor or blender with ⅛ cup heavy cream (scald the cream first) and 2 to 3 table-spoons unsalted butter. Process until smooth.

ROASTING whole is the easiest way to tenderize squash. If you can fit a squash into your oven, you can bake it whole. Just scrub it, puncture it in several places to allow hot air to vent, place it on a baking sheet (it will ooze juice that you don't want to bake on your oven), and put it in a 375°F oven for at least 45 minutes for a small squash, up to 1½ hours for a large one. Test with a knife or skewer, and when the flesh is tender, remove, let cool, then cut through the middle and remove the seeds and strings.

Preserving Cucurbits

Cucumbers don't freeze well; they contain too much water. But freezing is a perfect way to preserve summer and winter squash. Cut into halves, quarters, or chunks. Blanch for 3 to 4 minutes, then plunge into cold water. Drain fully, pack in airtight containers or freezer bags, and freeze. The squash will be mushy when thawed, but still usable in soups and stews. Or, puree squash (this is particularly useful for larger squash) and freeze for use in breads and muffins or as a soup thickener. Cucumbers do make the quintessential pickle, and zucchini pickles are a good way to preserve an overabundance of zucchini.

Cucurbit Nutrition

Cucumbers contain small amounts of vitamins A and C and are a good source of vitamin E. Cukes also provide fiber—some of which is lost if you remove the seeds—and fluids, since the flesh is about 95 percent water. Though they're more than 90 percent water, squash contain significant amounts of vitamins A and C, and some potassium and calcium. They're low in calories and high in fiber and fluids.

The nightshade family is a very diverse bunch: ornamental annual flowers like petunia, salpiglossis, and browallia; tobacco; poisons and hallucinogens (belladonna and jimsonweed); and some of our favorite vegetables, including tomatoes, peppers, eggplant, and potatoes (which you'll find in chapter 9). For a long time—up to the eighteenth century in some places—westerners didn't trust any of the family's members because of their relation to well-known poisons, and, in fact, some edible vegetables, like the eggplant and the potato, contain compounds that are toxic if the vegetable is eaten raw. And nightshades have been found to exacerbate arthritis in some people. But nightshades have become such an important—and delicious—part of our diet that few cuisines would be complete without them.

Eggplants, natives of Southeast Asia and possibly Africa, were particularly important ingredients in ancient Africa, Asia, and the Middle East, though they were avoided in Europe until the eighteenth century. Peppers are New World fruits; they were cultivated in South and Central America as early as 5,000 B.C.E. and spread quickly through Europe and Asia after Columbus's expeditions. Peppers are chameleons: Green ones turn red, yellow, and orange if allowed to stay on their vines for a few weeks; purple ones turn green. The color of the pepper indicates its ripeness. Most peppers are green in their immature stage, and though they keep better if picked green, they are not as sweet. Tomatoes originated in the Andes Mountains, but westerners wouldn't eat them for love (they were called love apples and considered to be highly aphrodisiac) or taste. Thomas Jefferson grew them at Monticello and tried to popularize them, but their poisonous reputation remained until the middle of the nineteenth century.

Most eggplant varieties taste pretty much the same; their quality is affected more by freshness and growing conditions than by place. Different shapes are associated with different regions. Asian eggplants are usually narrow and long, Italian ones are small and teardrop-shaped, and our standard U.S. eggplants are large and bottom-heavy. Eggplants come in many colors, from deep purple to the aptly named 'Applegreen,' white 'Caspar,' fluorescent lavender 'Neon,' and striped 'Zebra.' Tiny 'Bambino' and 'Little Finger' eggplants are perfect for pickling.

ALL ABOUT NIGHTSHADES

In the Field

Peppers split cleanly into two categories according to their level of a fiery element called capsaicin. Bell (sometimes called sweet) peppers contain very little of the capsaicin that makes peppers hot. Sweet peppers come in several shapes besides the boxy bells, including thin-skinned banana peppers and long, rectangular 'Cubanelles.' Most sweet peppers are great in salads, particularly those with thinner shells, while the heavier-walled bells are better for roasting and stuffing. Hot peppers contain levels of capsaicin that make them mildly spicy (like the Anaheim peppers that are used for chiles rellenos) to masochistically fiery ('Thai Hots' and 'Habaneros'). *Be careful* when dealing with fresh hot peppers; they can cause severe (though ultimately harmless) pain. Keep kids away from hot peppers.

Until just a few years ago, most of us knew only a few kinds of tomatoes: round, plum, and cherry. Breeders have been working on the tomato for years, but their goal has been more shippable, less perishable varieties, and many of the tomatoes that have resulted have had the texture of Styrofoam and a similar taste. Luckily, small farmers, independent breeders, and seed savers preserved some old-fashioned tomatoes, and we can now choose from a multitude of delicious heirloom tomatoes—the most famous is 'Brandywine,' but 'Cherokee Purple,' tiny 'Yellow Pear,' and 'Cosmonaut Volkov,' among others, deserve similar attention. And some relatively new hybrids, like heavenly 'Sungold' cherry tomatoes, have earned a place in the tomato spectrum as well.

All the nightshades hate cold weather and can't be planted out until days and nights are reliably frost-free (though they all prefer cool nights when they're beginning to grow). But once summer's heat sets in, they all produce prolifically for several weeks, until cooler weather reduces production. They will continue at lower levels until the first frost kills the plant. Peppers and eggplants grow on short, bushy plants. The inedible eggplant flower is a beautiful purple bell—a lovely addition to the garden, as is the heavy, beautifully shaped fruit that matures by early summer. Green (immature) peppers are usually ready by the first week of summer; they turn red and yellow a few weeks later, and by that time have to be picked and eaten quickly because they deteriorate soon after.

No one ever said it was easy to grow tomatoes. They host many diseases—especially the older varieties—and don't grow well unless they have the right combination of hot days, cool nights, and just enough water to keep from becoming waterlogged. And the juicier they are, the more fragile they are, so the best tomatoes are also the ones that split, rot, and fall apart. But they're worth it, aren't they?

Tomatoes should be brightly colored, be heavy for their size, and have no signs of splitting. Peppers will be light for their size, but should not have any brown patches or splits. Look for eggplants with fresh-looking caps and shiny, unblemished skin.

Eggplants become bitter with age and are very perishable. They should be stored in a cool, dry place and used within a day or two. If longer storage is necessary, place the eggplant in the refrigerator vegetable drawer. Green peppers will last in the crisper drawer of your refrigerator for one to two weeks. Don't wash them, because any moisture on them will promote rot. Storing them in a ventilated plastic bag keeps them dry. Red, yellow, and orange peppers will last only a few days. Always store your tomatoes at room temperature rather than in the refrigerator. Tomatoes will become red after they're picked, but they stop producing sugar; cold makes them start breaking those sugars down and robs them of flavor.

Eggplant is never eaten raw; cooking eliminates a toxic substance called solanine. When young, the skin of most eggplants is deliciously edible; older eggplants should be peeled. Since the flesh discolors rapidly, an eggplant should be cut just before using. Bitter, overripe fruit benefits from the ancient method of salting halves or slices and weighting them or placing them in a colander for 20 minutes before rinsing. The salt helps eliminate some of the acrid taste.

Eggplant can be prepared in a variety of ways, including baking, broiling, and frying. It does, however, have a spongelike capacity to soak up oil. You can reduce fat absorption by coating it well with a batter or crumb mixture. Salting eggplant as above, gently squeezing it, and patting it dry also makes it less absorbent. Soaking the eggplant in cold water for an hour or more, then patting it dry, has been found to work as well.

BAKING intensifies the flavor of eggplant. Prick all over with a fork and bake at 400°F for 40 to 50 minutes, until it is very soft. Let it cool before you cut it open and scrape out the pulp. Wrapping eggplant in aluminum foil before you put it in the oven makes it easier to handle.

BROILING OR GRILLING adds a delicious smokiness to eggplant. Slice the eggplant about ¼ inch thick. Brush the slices with olive oil and herbs. Place under the broiler or on the grill for 10 to 15 minutes, until tender, turning once. Eggplant makes great kabobs: Thread chunks on skewers, alone or with other vegetables, and broil or grill as above.

MICROWAVING can quickly provide eggplant puree for dips and casseroles. Make several deep cuts in the eggplant's skin and place it in a microwaveproof dish. Cover and cook on high for 3 to 4 minutes (more for a very large eggplant); turn over and cook for another 3 to 4 minutes. Let stand for 3 to 4 minutes, then scrape out the pulp. Slices can also be microwaved in a single layer on a microwave-safe plate; microwave uncovered for 6 to 8 minutes, then season.

SAUTÉING is the most traditional way of preparing eggplant. Slice thinly and sauté in hot oil until tender. Dipping in flour, egg, and then bread crumbs, or in any batter, makes frying faster and makes the eggplant less likely to soak up oil.

STEAMING quickly produces a soft pulp. Place the whole eggplant in an inch of water for 15 to 30 minutes. Scrape out the pulp and use in salads or dips.

STUFFING makes a meal out of a baked eggplant. Bake the eggplant for 20 minutes, then slice in half and scoop out the seeds. Stuff, then bake for an additional 20 to 30 minutes. (See Some Stuffings, page 164.)

ROASTING is an important first step in eggplant casseroles, dips, and stir-fries. To roast eggplant, brush slices with olive oil and herbs. Roast in a hot oven for 30 minutes until tender. Turn once during the roasting.

Peppers are tasty and nutritious raw—great in salads and as snacks; any cooking removes some of the nutrients. Here are the ways they are most often cooked:

ROASTING is a traditional way to bring out the sweetness of peppers and to loosen the skin so they may be peeled. To roast small hot peppers or any thin-walled peppers, heat a griddle and place the peppers on it. Press and flip with a pancake turner until they are lightly browned all over. When they are cool enough to handle, carefully (wear gloves—they are still hot!!!) remove the stems and seeds. To roast bell peppers, see page 163.

SAUTÉING adds flavor intensity to all kinds of peppers; just keep it brief. Cut the peppers into strips. Heat oil in a skillet until very hot (almost smoking). Add the peppers (throw in a hot pepper if you want) and sauté over high heat until they begin to color. Reduce the heat to medium, season with salt, cover the pan, and cook until the peppers are softened. You can then add a few tablespoons of vinegar, chopped garlic, or chopped fresh herbs (parsley, basil, mint, or oregano works well); toss over the heat for just a minute. Serve hot, cold, or at room temperature. Add olives, anchovies, or capers for more flavor.

STIR-FRYING takes advantage of the flavor and color of peppers to add excitement to a dish. Coat a skillet or wok with oil and heat until very hot; you may want to flavor the oil with onions and/or garlic. Add strips of pepper and toss rapidly, for 2 to 3 minutes.

STUFFING makes a half or a whole pepper a meal. To stuff bell peppers, slice off the top ½ inch, then scrape out the seeds and membranes. If the peppers won't stand, trim the bottoms, but don't make a hole or the juices will run out. If the peppers are very large, cut in half. Stuff (see Some Stuffings, page 164), then bake for 40 to 60 minutes.

Preparing Tomatoes

Tomatoes are delicious served raw, briefly cooked, or simmered for hours. They can be the star of a dish, one of many flavor components, or the sauce that gives definition to the recipe. Here are some ways to prepare them and preserve their identity:

BROILING OR GRILLING briefly introduces tomato slices to the heat and chars the surfaces of the slices while leaving the centers warm, sweet, and juicy. Cut the tomatoes into large slices (at least ½ inch thick; cut paste tomatoes in half). Brush with oil and herbs, and place under the broiler or on the grill for about 5 minutes.

ROASTING intensifies the tomato flavor and caramelizes the sugars in tomato halves. Place the tomatoes, cut side up, in a hot oven until the skin is charred but the flesh is still soft. To slow-roast, see page 163.

SWEATING is a gentle way to entice the juices from the tomatoes without any browning occurring. A good way to start a tomato sauce is to put sliced tomatoes into a saucepan with some unsalted butter, and about ½ teaspoon each of salt and sugar for each tomato used. Heat slowly, stirring constantly, until heated through, then lower the heat, cover, and continue cooking for 5 to 10 minutes, until the tomatoes have broken down. You can now season the tomatoes with herbs and add other vegetables to complete the sauce. For more about tomato sauces, see page 30.

Preserving Nightshades

Raw eggplant doesn't freeze well. If you can't use it quickly, prepare eggplant in dishes like moussaka, ratatouille, and eggplant dip and freeze in airtight containers. To freeze peppers, cut them into strips or bite-sized pieces (wash them first, and make sure they're completely dry before you put them in the freezer). They don't need blanching. Store in airtight containers or zippered plastic bags (they'll be soft but still good when thawed). Unpeeled roasted peppers can be frozen for up to one month; peel when thawed. Whole tomatoes freeze easily. Just put them in zippered plastic bags and place in the freezer. They're soft and a little mushy when they thaw but fine for sauces and purees. Or, make sauces or other dishes (like ratatouille) and freeze them. Drying is an excellent way to preserve tomatoes. Sun-drying really doesn't work in most North American climates, but home dehydrators will dry tomatoes perfectly with little work for you.

Nightshade Nutrition

Eggplant is not a great source of nutrients. But it's high in fiber and low in calories and so versatile that it can act as a base and an extender for foods that provide more vitamins and minerals. Peppers contain generous amounts of amino acids, potassium, and vitamins A and C and very few calories (just twenty-two in a large bell); red peppers have more vitamins A and C than green. Tomatoes are one of the best sources of lycopene, an antioxidant that helps prevent cell and tissue damage; cooking increases the amount of available lycopene. Recent studies have shown that consuming tomato sauces prevents many diseases. Tomatoes also provide beta-carotene, which is converted to vitamin A in the body, and substantial vitamin C. Use the seeds and the jellylike substance surrounding them; that's where most of the vitamin C is.

Cucumber and Yogurt

These two ingredients are combined in classic, cooling dips that originated in warm regions of the world. To make Greek *tzatziki,* mix 1 cup plain yogurt with 2 chopped garlic cloves, 1 large shredded cucumber, and 1 tablespoon lemon juice; season with salt and freshly milled black pepper and top with chopped fresh parsley. Indian *raitas* are a mellow accompaniment to spicy Indian foods: Combine 1 cup plain yogurt with 1 grated cucumber, 2 tablespoons finely chopped fresh mint, ½ teaspoon ground cumin and/or curry powder, and salt and freshly milled black pepper to taste. Create your own instant classics by mixing plain yogurt and cucumber with your favorite herbs, spices, vegetables, and even fruit. These cool concoctions can be thinned with milk or stock and pureed (or just stirred) for a hot or cold soup. Or, pour over hot or cold vegetables as a sauce or dressing.

TERITAR

MAKES 4 SERVINGS

The Philly Chile Company Farm CSA was named for the New Mexican chile 'Big Jim.' Inspired on a trip to the Southwest, Amanda McKutcheon, a chef, and Rob Ferber, manager of a farmers' market, started their farm in a New Jersey suburb of Philadelphia "to grow the freshest, finest-quality, organic produce available." They pick and distribute all their CSA's produce the same day and also sell sauces made from their chiles by mail order. This pesto-like dip is from Amanda's grandmother, who made it often on hot summer days.

½ cup chopped walnuts
1 garlic clove
2 medium cucumbers, peeled

¼ cup olive oil
1 teaspoon vinegar
½ teaspoon kosher salt

Combine the walnuts and garlic in a food processor fitted with the chopping blade; process to a paste.

Cut the cucumbers into large chunks; add to the walnut mixture and pulse until coarsely chopped. Add the oil, vinegar, and kosher salt; pulse until mixed but still somewhat chunky. Serve chilled or at cool room temperature.

Ulrike and Wendi Hilborn started Penn Cove Organics CSA in Oak Harbor, Washington, just before their first grandson, Matthew Ray, was born. "Grandma" Hilborn includes information about the baby in most of her *Cornucopia* newsletters, along with admonishments to "eat your vegetables," news of the fledgling farm's problems and successes, and recipes. She gets wonderful Greek recipes like this one from Thomas Soukakosis, owner of El Greco Restaurant.

GREEK ZUCCHINI CAKES

MAKES 24 CAKES

1 pound zucchini, grated
1 teaspoon kosher salt or ¾ teaspoon table salt
¾ cup crumbled feta cheese
1 large egg, lightly beaten
3 green onions, thinly sliced
3 tablespoons all-purpose flour
¼ cup chopped pine nuts

1 tablespoon chopped fresh dill, or 1 teaspoon dried
1½ teaspoons chopped fresh oregano, or ½ teaspoon dried
1 garlic clove, finely chopped
¼ teaspoon freshly milled black pepper
Olive oil

Combine the grated zucchini and kosher salt. Set aside for 5 minutes (no more, or it will be mush). Rinse in cold water and squeeze dry in a kitchen towel or press in a strainer or colander until dry.

Combine the cheese, egg, green onions, flour, pine nuts, dill, oregano, garlic, and pepper in a large bowl; fold in the zucchini. Form into 24 small cakes (about 2 tablespoons of mixture for each) and sauté in olive oil, turning once, until browned, about 3 minutes on each side. Serve immediately.

Meet the Farmers

Sunflower Fields Family Farm, Postville, Iowa

Neither Linda nor Michael Nash grew up on a farm, but Michael came to love farm life while working on a dairy farm near Rochester, New York, during college. The couple met while attending the Eastman School of Music. "After we were married and living here and there, we always talked about how, sometime, having a farm was something we'd like to do," Linda says. It took some time, but the couple has realized their dream. Sunflower Fields CSA is in its sixth season.

The couple started their search while Linda was an office manager for a group of surgeons and Michael was technical director for the Opera Theater of the University of Colorado. "It was a rat race," Linda recalls. They began buying newspapers from all over the upper Midwest as they scanned classified ads for land.

They purchased their 250-acre farm in rural Iowa for the same amount of money that they sold their home on 1½ acres in Colorado. Linda is particularly happy with the generous size of their farm, which allows them to rotate crops in a seven-year cycle so that they do not deplete the soil with any one vegetable. The farm has about twenty-five acres in production at any one time. Linda and Michael intentionally sought out a larger farm that would enable them to farm more responsibly rather than needing to keep all the land in production at all times. "We said whatever happens, let's get enough land to be able to go fallow, rotate, and cover-crop and not just pound, pound, pound, the soil," Linda recalls.

Unfortunately, even in Iowa, much of the fresh produce is shipped in long-distance from California, Linda says. That means hardiness, not taste, is the deciding factor when the far-off farms decide what varieties to plant. Small local farms can give more consideration to consumers' taste buds because they don't have to worry about the great distance and time that separates them from their customers.

Of the several recipes for heirloom tomato salad that were submitted for this book, this version, from Ross Browne, executive chef of Absinthe Brasserie and Bar in San Francisco, stood out for its flavor and simplicity. Chef Browne told us that he makes this only when local tomatoes are at their peak. He tries to include four or five varieties of different sizes, shapes, and colors, and never refrigerates the tomatoes, because that reduces their flavor. He added that it is important to dress the salad only moments before serving so that the vinegar doesn't draw the juice from the tomatoes, and also suggested, "If the tomatoes are really good, you may not want to add vinegar at all, just a few drops of your favorite extra-virgin olive oil."

HEIRLOOM TOMATOES WITH FRESH HERBS, TOASTED PINE NUTS, AND TAPENADE TOAST POINTS

MAKES 6 SERVINGS

Tapenade (recipe follows)
2 pounds assorted heirloom tomatoes
6 white or whole wheat bread slices, crusts removed
Extra-virgin olive oil
Balsamic or red wine vinegar
Sea salt and freshly milled black pepper
2 tablespoons chopped assorted fresh herbs and blossoms
2 tablespoons pine nuts, toasted (see Note)

Prepare the tapenade.

Cut the larger tomatoes into slices, removing the stem ends; cut the smaller tomatoes into wedges; if using cherry or 'Sweet 100' tomatoes, leave them whole. Divide the tomatoes among 6 salad plates.

Cut the bread slices diagonally in half and toast. Spread the tapenade evenly over the toast points in a thin layer, covering completely to the edges.

Season the tomatoes with oil, vinegar, and sea salt and pepper to taste; sprinkle with the herbs and pine nuts. Place 2 toast points on each salad and serve.

NOTE: Spread the pine nuts on an ungreased tray and toast in a 350°F oven or in a toaster oven just until they are aromatic, 6 to 8 minutes.

TAPENADE: Combine 1 cup pitted, rinsed Niçoise olives, 2 tablespoons orange juice, 1½ tablespoons grated orange peel, 1 tablespoon whole almonds chopped lightly and toasted, 1 tablespoon olive oil, 1 chopped garlic clove, and ⅓ teaspoon Pernod, if desired, in a food processor fitted with the chopping blade. Pulse until coarsely chopped.

Salsas

"*Salsa*" is simply the Mexican word for sauce, but the term has come to stand for a rhythmic form of music and dance and a kicky little salad. The salsas we eat can be made from mostly raw vegetables (*salsa cruda*) or cooked vegetables (*salsa verde* generally includes cooked tomatillos, tomatoes, and chiles). Most recipes call for at least a little hot pepper, but salsas don't have to rely on heat to be interesting; the following are just a few of the hundreds of combinations that we've found:

Corn and Greens: 5 cups shredded sharp greens (arugula, watercress, radicchio), kernels from 3 ears of corn, ¼ cup cider vinegar, and 1 to 2 small hot peppers, minced.

Jicama-Onion: About 8 ounces diced jicama; 8 ounces diced Vidalia onions; ¼ cup white or cider vinegar, 3 tablespoons chopped fresh cilantro; 2 to 3 garlic cloves; minced; and 2 (or more) hot peppers, minced.

Red Pepper: 2 red bell peppers, sliced; 1 medium cucumber, chopped; 2 green onions, chopped; 3 tablespoons chopped fresh cilantro; and 1 small hot pepper, minced.

Watermelon and Red Onion: 2 large watermelon slices, cut into ½-inch chunks; 1 large red onion, diced; 1 bunch fresh cilantro, chopped; and ½ cup balsamic vinegar.

Avocado-Tomato: 2 tomatoes, diced; 1 small avocado, in chunks; 2 tablespoons chopped fresh cilantro; 1 tablespoon cider vinegar; and 2 teaspoons lime juice.

This recipe comes from Miki Knowles, a consulting chef and recipe developer for B&W Quality Growers, a family-owned farm based in Fellsmere, Florida, that specializes in growing arugula and watercress. Miki, who is also a food stylist, works with many small and organic farmers from whom she often buys produce for photo shoots. "A lot of people say organic food doesn't look good," Miki says, "but I find that the farms I deal with really take such care in raising their crops that they have the most beautiful vegetables." For this salad, she suggests roasting your own peppers, because she finds most jarred roasted peppers to be less than flavorful. After blackened peppers are removed from the oven, Miki recommends that they be placed in a plastic container or paper bag to encourage them to sweat. Once they're cooled, the skin peels right off.

ROASTED PEPPER AND ARUGULA SALAD

MAKES 4 SERVINGS

2 large red bell peppers
3 tablespoons olive oil
1 teaspoon sugar
1 teaspoon Dijon mustard
1 garlic clove, chopped

4 to 5 ounces arugula, rinsed, drained, trimmed, and crisped
1 small head radicchio, separated, rinsed, drained, and crisped

Preheat a grill or the broiler; grill or broil the peppers until fairly blackened. Transfer the peppers into a plastic container or a paper bag (closed tight); set aside to cool to room temperature.

Meanwhile, combine the oil, sugar, mustard, and garlic in a small jar and shake well.

Break the arugula and radicchio into pieces and combine in a large bowl. When the peppers have cooled, remove and discard the skins, seeds, and cores. Coarsely chop the peppers and toss with the arugula and radicchio.

Shake the dressing well; drizzle over the salad and toss. Divide among 4 salad plates and serve.

Pulp Facts

No one ever said eggplant pulp was pretty, but it's a beautiful base for spreads and salads. To make it, just puncture a large eggplant in a few places and wrap it loosely in aluminum foil. Place it in a 400°F oven until it's soft and mushy—it's usually ready in about an hour, but longer baking won't hurt it. Let it cool completely, then scrape all the flesh off the purple skin. You'll get about 1½ cups of pulp from a medium eggplant. Add whatever other vegetables and herbs you like—the eggplant's mild taste and pleasant texture blends and binds other ingredients.

Baba Ghanoush: Add to mashed eggplant pulp 2 tablespoons tahini (ground sesame see paste), 2 tablespoons lemon juice, 1 tablespoon olive oil, 1 tablespoon chopped fresh cilantro or parsley, 2 garlic cloves, minced (mashed or pureed roasted garlic is even better), 1 teaspoon cumin seeds, and salt and ground red pepper to taste. Mix well and serve with pita.

Thai Eggplant Dip: Combine mashed eggplant pulp, 3 to 4 garlic cloves, chopped, and 1 tablespoon peeled minced fresh ginger; puree in a food processor or blender until smooth. Add 2 tablespoons rice wine vinegar, 2 tablespoons sesame oil, 2 tablespoons soy sauce, and 2 tablespoons chopped fresh cilantro or parsley. Add salt and red pepper to taste.

Abu Ghanoush: Instead of mashing the eggplant pulp, chop it roughly and toss it with 1 bell pepper, finely sliced; 2 to 3 medium tomatoes, finely sliced; and 1 small onion, finely sliced. In a small bowl, mix the juice of 1 lemon or lime, 1 tablespoon olive oil, 1 tablespoon chopped fresh parsley or cilantro, 2 garlic cloves, minced, 1 teaspoon ground cumin, a pinch of ground red pepper, and salt to taste. Combine with the eggplant mixture.

Meet the Farmers

Green Market Farm, New Salem, Massachusetts

Karen Wallman and her husband, John, are both city kids by birth but farmers at heart. Karen, for one, always had a feeling that farming was in her future. But her interest in gardening didn't mean automatic success. When she planted her first garden, she was in her twenties. She was so excited that her radishes were growing at all that she let them grow, and grow, and grow. By the time she harvested them, "You could have whittled them like wood," she recalls. But she didn't give up. Karen, an artist, grew even more inspired by the beauty of farming when she and her husband, a chiropractor, moved out to a relatively rural section of northern Long Island in New York State. By 1989, they'd decided it was time to get their own land, so they bought just under three acres in Massachusetts. They operate a buying club that distributes organic produce from a wholesale distributor, as well as a retail shop where Karen sometimes sells her artwork along with her homemade jams and mustards. They added their CSA to the mix two years ago.

Pumpkins need so much water and manure that Karen sees them as a kind of guilty pleasure, especially when she considers most end up on doorsteps as seasonal ornaments. But at the end of the season it's all worthwhile. When she's hunted out the dozens of beautiful orange orbs from their hiding places under the large green leaves, she can't help but fall in love with the crop yet again. "Pumpkins are magical," says Karen.

Green Market Farm is an organic farm that is saving up to become certified organic one day. Unlike many small farmers, Karen believes the new federal organic standards may one day benefit her. "It gives me something I can strive for," says Karen. "Without consumers, we're just growing this stuff for ourselves. What the standards will do is create customer trust."

GAZPACHO

MAKES 8 SERVINGS

Frances Walker of Eatwell Farm in Winters, California, is a gazpacho maven but points out that gazpachos are hard to pin down—there are more than thirty recipes for this soup in Spain, where it originated. Frances often adds grated summer squash of different colors—she grates the squash as well as the tomatoes, onions, and cucumbers because that provides more juice as well as a better texture. But she throws peppers and garlic into the blender, because they chop better that way (the garlic goes in first, alone). Instead of cutting bread for croutons, she just puts big chunks at the bottom of the bowl. And she throws a few ice cubes into the soup because it cools it down quickly for immediate eating and thins down heavier gazpachos. This gazpacho was contributed by a CSA member.

9 large vine-ripened tomatoes
2 medium cucumbers, peeled, seeded, and chopped
1 medium red onion, chopped
1 bell pepper, chopped
⅓ cup olive oil
6 tablespoons red wine vinegar, or to taste

3 garlic cloves, finely chopped
1 to 2 jalapeño peppers, finely chopped
Salt and freshly milled black pepper
¼ cup thinly sliced fresh basil, cilantro, or parsley (optional)

Core the tomatoes and dip into boiling water for about 10 seconds to loosen the skin. Place the tomatoes in ice water to cool, then slip off their skins. Cut the tomatoes in half crosswise and squeeze out the juice and seeds into a strainer over a bowl. Reserve the juice and discard the seeds. Puree half of the tomatoes in a food processor or blender. Coarsely chop the remaining tomatoes.

Combine the pureed and chopped tomatoes in a bowl and add the reserved juice. Stir in the cucumbers, red onion, bell pepper, oil, vinegar, garlic, and jalapeño peppers. Season with salt and black pepper to taste. Chill for at least 1 hour before serving. Sprinkle the fresh herb over the bowls for garnish, if desired.

Heirlooms

The term "heirloom" has become common in culinary circles lately, though it doesn't have an exact or accepted definition. Heirloom vegetables are the ones that were grown before breeders forgot about trying to find the best taste and started hybridizing for transportability, ease of growing, uniformity, and pest resistance. Some people say that heirlooms have to be at least fifty years old, and many of them are much older; we can trace some of our favorite seeds back to colonial times; and dinosaur kale may go back even further than that.

One attribute that most heirlooms share is that they're open-pollinated—that is, their seeds produce exact replicas of themselves. Many modern hybrids are unstable; if you save and plant their seeds, you'll get one of their parents, or a less favorable combination.

Let's not forget that not all progress is bad. Some recent hybrids, like 'Sungold' cherry tomatoes, can beat any of our grandmothers' versions for taste. And resistance to disease and pests is a very useful attribute, especially for organic farms. (We're not referring to genetically modified varieties—for more information about those, see page 262.) Some of the older varieties, though delicious, are so prone to pests that growing them without pesticides is practically impossible above the home-garden, pick-off-every-bug-by-hand scale.

But we don't need every one of our vegetables to be perfectly formed and blemish-free; huge, misshapen heirloom tomatoes, full of juice and flavor, deserve a place in our markets and at our tables. We don't want to lose our vegetable heritage, and by buying heirloom vegetables from our CSAs and farmers' markets, we're keeping them in the gene pool so that we can enjoy them and whatever hybrids can be bred from them in the future.

There are thousands of heirloom vegetables, including the ones whose seeds your grandmother saves from year to year, but whose names she has forgotten. Here are just a few: 'Early Jersey Wakefield' cabbage, teardrop-shaped, pale green, delicate flavor; 'Scarlet Runner' beans, grown by Thomas Jefferson; 'Chioggia' striped beets, an Italian heirloom; 'Cherries Jubiliee' potatoes, bite-sized, red-skinned, easy to grow; 'Jacob's Cattle' dried beans, which can be stored for months; 'Brandywine' tomatoes, which are reputed to have the best taste in the world and were at the forefront of the heirloom revolution, as well as 'Cherokee Purple,' which have black streaks and an even more interesting taste than Brandywine.

BUTTERNUT SQUASH AND CIDER BISQUE

MAKES 6 SERVINGS

Donna Karch of Mountain Melody Gardens in Palenville, New York, grows flowers that she sells through CSAs and farmers' markets. Her flowers are all organically grown; many of us don't realize how much pesticides and synthetic fertilizer are introduced into the environment by flower growers, especially those in unregulated countries. Donna is also a wonderful cook; this soup was brought to a Carnegie Hill/Yorkville CSA potluck and devoured in minutes.

4 tablespoons (½ stick) unsalted
   butter
2 cups onions, diced
4 teaspoons curry powder
2 medium butternut squash

2 apples
3 cups vegetable or chicken stock
1 cup apple cider
Salt and freshly milled black pepper

Melt the butter in a large kettle and sauté the onions and curry powder over very low heat for about 25 minutes.

Meanwhile, peel the squash and apples and cut them into chunks (see Note). Add the squash, apples, and stock to the kettle and simmer for 25 minutes. Mash the solids with a potato masher or transfer the contents of the kettle to a blender and puree (depending on how much texture you like).

Return pureed bisque to the kettle; add the cider and season to taste with salt and pepper.

NOTE: If you find the squash too hard to cut, bake it in a 400°F oven for about 20 minutes before peeling and cubing it.

Salad Stuff

Other than lettuce, tomatoes are probably the most common ingredient of salads. Here are a few international classics:

Salad Caprese: Overlap slices of ripe tomato and fresh mozzarella. Whisk together 3 table-spoons olive oil, 2 tablespoons balsamic vinegar, 1 tablespoon finely chopped fresh basil, and salt and freshly milled black pepper to taste. Drizzle the dressing over the salad and garnish with whole basil leaves.

Israeli Salad: Combine 1 cup each finely chopped cucumber and finely chopped tomato. Mix ¼ cup cider vinegar with 2 tablespoons vegetable oil and 1 tablespoon finely chopped fresh pars-ley. Toss the dressing with the salad and add salt and freshly milled black pepper to taste.

Greek Salad: Combine chunks of tomato, red onion, bell pepper, and cucumber in a salad bowl. Sprinkle ½ cup crumbled feta cheese over the salad. Dress with olive oil, and white wine vinegar mixed with chopped fresh oregano. Garnish with ½ cup sliced Greek olives.

Latino Salad: Overlap slices of tomato, red onion, and avocado. Whisk together 3 tablespoons lime juice, 3 tablespoons olive oil, 2 tablespoons chopped fresh cilantro, and salt and freshly milled black pepper to taste. Drizzle the dressing over the salad.

Tuscan Bread Salad: Cut 6 slices of stale bread into chunks. Soak the bread in milk or water for about 30 seconds, then press gently in a colander and set aside for 30 minutes to drain. Mean-while, chop 3 tomatoes and cut a red onion into chunks; combine with 2 tablespoons finely chop-ped fresh basil. Combine with the bread and toss gently with a vinaigrette dressing.

TACOS DE CALABACITAS A LA MEXICANA

MEXICAN-STYLE ZUCCHINI TACOS

MAKES ABOUT 6 CUPS,
FILLING ABOUT 24 TACOS,
SERVING 6 AS A CASUAL MEAL

Rick Bayless, chef/owner of Frontera Grill/Topolobampo Restaurants in Chicago and host of public television's *Mexico—One Plate at a Time,* was the first chef to contribute a recipe for this book. He told us that his goal as a chef and restaurateur is "to support the principles of sustainability of our planet by buying organically or naturally raised foods, working with local farmers, thoughtfully using (and reusing) resources, and disposing of waste; to carry the principles of sustainability into our lives and those of our coworkers by developing realistic performance expectations."

1 ½ tablespoons vegetable oil
1 medium white onion, chopped
1 pound (6 to 8 plum or 2 medium-large round) ripe tomatoes, roughly chopped, or ⅔ of a 28-ounce can good-quality whole tomatoes in juice, drained
2 garlic cloves, finely chopped
2 large fresh poblano chiles
Kernels from 1 large ear fresh corn (about 1 cup)
4 medium (about 1 ½ pounds) zucchini, or use the Mexican round or teardrop-shaped light green calabacitas, cut into ½-inch cubes (about 5 cups of cubes)

Leaves from 1 sprig fresh epazote, roughly chopped or 3 tablespoons chopped fresh cilantro
⅔ cup homemade crema, crème fraîche, or heavy (whipping) cream
Salt
½ cup (about 2 ounces) Mexican queso fresco or other crumbly fresh cheese like salted pressed farmer's cheese or feta
24 fresh, warm corn tortillas

Preparing the flavoring base: Measure the oil into a large (12-inch) skillet set over medium-high heat. Add the onion and cook, stirring frequently, until richly browned, about 8 minutes. While the onion is cooking, coarsely puree the tomatoes in a food processor or blender. Add the garlic to the browned onion, cook for 1 minute, stirring, then add the tomatoes. Reduce the heat to medium-low, cover the skillet, and cook, stirring occasionally, for 5 minutes. Remove from the heat.

Roasting the chiles: Roast the poblanos directly over a gas flame or on a baking sheet 4 inches below a very hot broiler, turning regularly until the skin

Future Classics

We take certain vegetable preparations for granted: mashed potatoes, pickled cucumbers, coleslaws. The following creations aren't staples yet, but if enough people try them, they will be soon!

Roasted Peppers: Place bell peppers—whole or cut in half (remove the seeds if you're cutting in half)—under the broiler or over an open flame until the skin is blackened. (If roasting whole, turn them often.) Then slip off the skins (placing blackened peppers in a paper bag for 15 minutes before peeling makes the skins come off more easily). They're now soft and sweet.

Slow-Roasted Tomatoes: Cut tomatoes into ¾-inch slices and place them on a baking sheet. (Line it with aluminum foil or parchment paper—or face a difficult cleanup!) Sprinkle the tomatoes with a pinch of brown sugar, salt, and pepper; drizzle with olive oil; then sprinkle with chopped fresh herbs (basil is best). Bake at 250°F for at least 3 hours, until the tomatoes are shriveled; let cool before serving. Slow-roasting concentrates tomato flavor; even mediocre tomatoes taste good when prepared this way, and great tomatoes turn so sweet, they taste like candy.

Add a vinaigrette to either of the above, and they're a delicious side dish. Puree that side dish, and you have a great dip; thin with milk, cream, or stock, and you have a soup.

has blistered and blackened on all sides, about 5 minutes for an open flame, about 10 minutes for the broiler. Cover with a kitchen towel and let stand for 5 minutes. Rub off the blackened skins, then pull out the stems and seed-pods. Rinse briefly to remove stray seeds and bits of skin. Slice into ¼-inch strips.

Finishing the dish: Uncover the skillet and raise the heat to medium-high. Stir in the poblanos, corn, zucchini, epazote (or cilantro), and the *crema* (or one of its stand-ins). Cook, stirring frequently, until the zucchini is crisp-tender and the liquid has thickened enough to coat the vegetables nicely, about 8 minutes. Taste and season with salt, usually about 1 teaspoon. Serve in a decorative bowl, sprinkle with the crumbled cheese, and pass the hot tortillas separately for do-it-yourself tacos.

Some Stuffings

These mixtures can be used to stuff hollowed-out peppers, eggplants, large summer squash (especially pattypans), even onions. This is enough stuffing for about 4 small bell peppers, 2 large squash, or 4 small pattypans (about 4 servings). After preparing the stuffing, arrange the vegetables to be filled in a baking pan, stuff, and bake in a 375°F oven for 45 minutes to 1 hour, until the stuffing is browned.

Fresh Vegetables and Cheese: Toss 2 chopped tomatoes, 1 diced medium onion, ½ cup chopped fresh basil, 2 minced garlic cloves, and salt and freshly milled black pepper to taste. Sauté briefly in 2 tablespoons olive oil. Combine with 2 cups cheese (grated mozzarella or Cheddar or ricotta, or a mixture). Top with grated Parmesan.

Sausage and Squash: Mix 12 ounces sweet Italian sausage (casings removed), 1 cup coarsely grated zucchini, ¼ cup finely chopped onion, ¼ cup fine dried bread crumbs, 1 small egg, 3 tablespoons minced fresh parsley, ½ teaspoon freshly milled black pepper, ½ teaspoon salt, ½ teaspoon minced fresh rosemary.

Spicy Chicken: Combine 3 cooked and diced chicken breast halves, 6 ounces cream cheese, 2 diced green onions, 2 minced garlic cloves, and 1 diced small hot pepper in a medium bowl; stir to blend. Add ½ cup grated cheese (Monterey Jack, mozzarella, Swiss), 1 large egg, and 2 tablespoons heavy cream; stir to combine. Season with salt, freshly milled black pepper, chili powder, and cumin to taste.

Rice and Beef: Combine a 28-ounce can tomatoes, 8 ounces ground beef, 1½ cups cooked brown rice, 1 diced small onion, 1 large egg, 2 minced garlic cloves, 1 teaspoon chili powder, 1 teaspoon dried oregano, and a dash of Worcestershire sauce. Add, as desired, 1 cup sautéed mushrooms or other vegetables; other herbs; hot peppers.

Cheese and Greens: Heat 2 tablespoons olive oil in a skillet; sauté 1 chopped small onion and 3 minced garlic cloves. Add 4 cups chopped greens; sauté until softened. Combine with 2 cups grated cheese. Season with salt, freshly milled black pepper, and herbs.

This recipe, contributed by Scott Mathieson of Laguna Farms, Sebastopol, California, is a complete meal in one dish. It's easily adaptable to whatever vegetables are in season, and you can add different herbs to the tomato sauce to vary the flavor. The rice forms a substantial base—tamp the rice down gently—and the cheese topping crusts beautifully during the baking time. It also freezes and reheats well.

PICANTE ZUCCHINI

MAKES 6 SERVINGS

1½ pounds tomatoes, coarsely chopped
1 (6-ounce) can tomato paste
3 garlic cloves, finely chopped
1 tablespoon chopped fresh cilantro
   or chives
1 hot pepper, chopped, or ground red
   pepper to taste

1 teaspoon finely chopped fresh
   rosemary
Salt
3 medium zucchini, sliced ¼ inch thick
Olive oil
2 cups cooked rice
2 cups grated Cheddar cheese

Combine the tomatoes, tomato paste, garlic, cilantro, hot pepper, and rosemary in a medium saucepan. Cook over low heat until the tomatoes are very tender, about 30 minutes. Add a little water, if necessary, to make 2 cups. Taste and add salt.

Meanwhile, sauté the zucchini in olive oil until tender and lightly browned, about 3 minutes on each side. Remove to paper towels to drain.

Preheat the oven to 350°F. Oil a 2-quart casserole or baking dish. Spread the rice evenly in the bottom of the dish; cover with the zucchini slices. Pour the tomato sauce over the top and sprinkle with the cheese. Bake for about 45 minutes, or until bubbly and browned.

AUTUMN SQUASH PASTA

MAKES 8 SIDE-DISH SERVINGS

This easy-to-make dish, by Jenni and Pete Cosenza, was a hit at one of the Carnegie Hill/Yorkville CSA's potluck suppers last year. Even the children came back for seconds. This is a nice side dish to accompany a simple grilled chicken, though it may be eaten as a main course as well.

3 to 4 pounds acorn or butternut
  squash
1 pound ziti or penne
½ cup olive oil
2 tablespoons unsalted butter
2 large leeks, cleaned and coarsely
  chopped
½ small onion, chopped

1 garlic clove, coarsely chopped
½ to 1 teaspoon coarse sea salt,
  or more to taste
Freshly milled black pepper
½ cup dry white wine or water
⅓ cup grated Parmesan cheese
1 tablespoon chopped fresh parsley

Preheat the oven to 350°F. Cut the squash in half; scoop out and discard the seeds. Place the squash, cut side down, in 1 inch of water in a 13- by 9-inch glass baking dish. Bake for 45 to 50 minutes, until tender. Set aside just until cool enough to handle, then scoop the squash from the shells.

Meanwhile, cook the pasta in boiling salted water for 2 to 3 minutes less than the cooking time on the package; drain and set aside.

Heat the oil and butter in a large pot over low heat. Add the leeks, onion, garlic, sea salt, and pepper. Sauté until the onion is translucent and the leeks have become pliable, making sure the garlic does not burn. Add the squash and wine, stirring until a thick sauce forms. Fold in the cooked pasta; taste and adjust the seasonings. Spoon into the same glass baking dish; sprinkle with the cheese.

Bake for 20 to 30 minutes, until the cheese browns; sprinkle with the parsley and serve hot.

Corporate Tomatoes

Here's how Leigh Hauter of Bull Run Mountain Organic Farm, The Plains, Virginia, instructs his CSA members on handling tomatoes:

"Corporate tomatoes, the ones that you buy in the grocery stores, are a completely different creature from what we grow. First, corporate tomatoes aren't grown around here. Almost all of America's summer tomatoes originate in California, in the fabulously polluted San Joaquin Valley, and are then shipped across the country.

"And how is something as delicate as a tomato transported all of those thousands of miles? Simple. They are picked green and often treated with a gas to make them turn red. And why, you might ask, would anyone pick their tomatoes green (unless they wanted fried green tomatoes)? The answer: Tomatoes picked green are firmer, less juicy, more capable of bouncing around in a box, and, in the store, of being picked up and squeezed. It takes an awful lot to make them go squish. Corporate tomatoes have what homegrown tomatoes don't have. They have 'shelf life.'

"Fresh, picked-this-morning tomatoes are different. They are full of juice. The fruit walls are tender. If they are given a squeeze, they go squish. And if you put them in a box and ship them halfway around the world, what comes out at the other end is tomato juice, not tomatoes. Local, homegrown tomatoes are a completely different creature from those corporate vegetables. They are full of juice. They can't handle being squeezed.

"So, to make the story short, when you are picking out your tomatoes, just look at them, and touch only the tomatoes you are going to put in your bag. And if, by chance, you don't particularly like that tomato after picking it up, put it in your bag anyway, and just take another one."

SQUASH "PIZZA"

MAKES 4 SERVINGS

Mike Kuhn, a former volunteer for Angelic Organics CSA and a Chicago-based chef, taught classes for the farm that were designed to help shareholders learn to cook and manage the vegetables they received every week. Mike said that the challenges of CSA cooking are similar to the so-called "market-basket test" popular in cooking schools, where students must rely on their ingenuity to cook up a box of ingredients on the spot. He gave this recipe to Maura Webber, to accompany an article she wrote on his class. The piece, "Organics Find Audience in Pilsen: Touched by Angelic," was published in the *Chicago Sun-Times* on June 7, 2000.

2 organic green zucchini, quartered
    lengthwise
2 organic yellow squash, quartered
    lengthwise
1/4 cup olive oil
Salt and freshly milled black pepper
1 organic tomato, diced

1 Spanish onion, diced
Leaves from 4 fresh thyme sprigs,
    chopped, or 1/2 teaspoon dried
    thyme
1/4 cup fresh basil leaves, washed, dried,
    and chopped
1 cup grated Cheddar cheese

Preheat the oven to 400°F. Oil an ovenproof baking dish.

Alternate the zucchini and yellow squash, cut side up, in the dish. Drizzle with the oil and season with salt and pepper. Sprinkle the tomato, onion, thyme, and basil over the zucchini and squash; top with the cheese.

Bake, uncovered, for about 20 minutes, or until the cheese is melted and the zucchini and squash soften.

The Cook College Student Organic Farm at New Jersey's Rutgers University is the nation's largest organic farm managed by university students. For the past seven years, students have cultivated and maintained three acres of land and provided food for its 120 members and the Elijah's Promise Soup Kitchen. Students manage all aspects of the CSA and coordinate produce donations and deliveries. The program promotes healthy cooking; this classic Greek recipe uses low-fat cottage cheese instead of cream in its custard, but you'll be surprised at how creamy and tasty the result is.

EGGPLANT PASTITSIO

MAKES 4 SERVINGS

2 tablespoons vegetable oil
1 large eggplant, peeled and cut into
　1-inch cubes
1/2 cup chopped onions
1/2 cup tomato paste
1/2 cup dry white wine
1/2 teaspoon salt
1/2 teaspoon dried oregano

1/4 teaspoon ground cinnamon
　(optional)
1/4 teaspoon ground allspice (optional)
4 large eggs, beaten
1 cup low-fat cottage cheese
3 tablespoons grated Parmesan cheese
2 cups cooked elbow macaroni

Heat the oil in a large skillet over medium heat. Add the eggplant and onions. Cook, stirring frequently, for 10 minutes. Reduce the heat to low. Stir in the tomato paste, wine, salt, oregano, cinnamon, if using, and allspice, if using. Cover and simmer, stirring occasionally, for 15 minutes.

Preheat the oven to 350°F. Spray an 8-inch square baking dish with vegetable cooking spray.

Combine the eggs, cottage cheese, and Parmesan cheese in a small bowl. Spread 1 cup of the eggplant mixture in the bottom of the baking dish. Top with the macaroni, then the cheese mixture, and then the remaining eggplant mixture. Bake, uncovered, for 30 minutes.

VEGETABLE MOUSSAKA

MAKES 4 SERVINGS

This recipe comes from Steve Waxman of Carnegie Hill/Yorkville CSA in Manhattan; he is one of our favorite sources for recipes for our newsletter. Steve added these tips: "We consistently receive a high quantity and quality of eggplant. Other than baking the whole eggplant for a Middle Eastern–style salad, this is our favorite way to prepare it for ready use during the week."

Olive oil
Freshly milled black pepper
2 medium or 1 large eggplant, peeled and cut diagonally into ¼-inch-thick slices
4 green onions, thinly sliced
3 garlic cloves, thinly sliced
1 tablespoon unsalted butter
2 medium baking potatoes, thinly sliced

½ tablespoon chopped fresh oregano, or ½ teaspoon dried
½ teaspoon salt
1 teaspoon garam masala, or to taste
4 ounces goat cheese, crumbled
2 medium tomatoes, sliced ¼ inch thick
½ cup plain low-fat yogurt
2 tablespoons chopped fresh parsley
¼ teaspoon lemon juice

Heat ½ tablespoon oil and about ⅛ teaspoon pepper in a heavy skillet over medium heat. Place the eggplant slices in the skillet, making sure that the surface of each slice makes full contact with the pan. Let the eggplant cook on each side for about 3 minutes, periodically pressing on each slice with a spatula. Set aside the cooked slices and repeat, adding oil and a bit more pepper as necessary (see Note), until all the eggplant has been cooked. In the same skillet, sauté the green onions and garlic in 1 tablespoon oil for about 2 minutes.

Preheat the oven to 350°F. Spread the butter around the inside of a 9-inch square baking dish. Place a layer of the potatoes and sprinkle with half of the oregano, half of the salt, and ⅛ teaspoon pepper. Add half of the eggplant, sprinkle with half of the garam masala and half of the goat cheese, and top with half of the tomato slices. Next add the onion-and-garlic mixture. Then, repeat the potato, eggplant, cheese, and tomato layers. Bake, uncovered, for about 45 minutes, or until the potatoes are tender. Test occasionally for doneness with a sharp knife.

Meanwhile, prepare the yogurt sauce. Combine the yogurt, parsley, and lemon juice in a small bowl and refrigerate. Serve the moussaka topped with yogurt sauce.

NOTE: Eggplant absorbs a lot of liquid, so do not use too much oil at a time. You can also add a liquid such as wine, beer, or stock if the pan is getting too hot and you don't want to add more oil.

EASY PASTA FRESCA

MAKES 8 SERVINGS

Lynn Thor of Whistle-Stop Gardens in Tunnel, New York, raises beef as well as vegetables, but many of her favorite recipes, like this one, are vegetarian. Her favorite tomatoes for this sauce are Brandywines. Lynn says that sliced fennel, zucchini, or summer squash are good optional additions to the recipe. Besides serving it over pasta or rice, she uses this sauce to top pizza.

4 small eggplants, peeled and cut into
 1-inch cubes
2 red bell peppers, cut into 1-inch
 pieces
1 large onion, coarsely chopped
4 or more large garlic cloves, peeled
Olive oil

2 to 3 large beefsteak tomatoes,
 peeled, seeded, and chopped
1/4 cup chopped fresh basil
1/4 cup chopped fresh parsley
1/2 teaspoon balsamic vinegar
Salt and freshly milled black pepper
8 servings hot cooked pasta or rice
Parmesan cheese

Preheat the oven to 400°F. Combine the eggplant, peppers, onion, and garlic with enough olive oil to coat. Spread in an oiled shallow baking dish and roast for about 45 minutes, stirring every 10 minutes or so, until nicely caramelized.

Mash together the tomatoes, basil, parsley, roasted garlic cloves, and balsamic vinegar; fold into the remaining roasted vegetables. Do not cook; taste, and add salt and pepper.

Serve at room temperature, or slightly warmed, over pasta or rice, or use as a pizza topping. Pass your favorite grated cheese (Parmesan or feta is excellent).

TOMATILLO TACO CASSEROLE

MAKES 4 SERVINGS

Clay Brook Farm, a thirty-six-acre certified organic farm in Jericho, Vermont, has been farmed intermittently over the last 140 years and was being used to raise sheep before Bob Hill and Laury Shea bought it in 1997. Bob and Laury grow a wide variety of vegetables and flowers, which they sell to restaurants, natural food stores, and florists, and at local farmers' markets. In 1999, they started the CSA component of their farm, and it's grown to include more than seventy-five families. This recipe was contributed by member Carol Lee Mason.

1 pound ground turkey, beef, or soy substitute
1 small onion, chopped
1 to 2 small hot peppers, chopped (optional)
1 garlic clove, minced
6 cups lightly crushed tortilla chips
2 cups cooked black or kidney beans

1 ½ cups halved small tomatillos (see Note)
Salt and freshly milled black pepper
1 cup grated Cheddar or Monterey Jack cheese
1 cup sour cream
1 cup prepared salsa

Preheat the oven to 350°F. Lightly oil the bottom of a 13- by 9-inch baking pan.

Brown the meat in a large, heavy skillet over medium heat. Add the onion, hot peppers, if using, and garlic; cook until tender.

Spread the tortilla chips in the bottom of the baking pan. Top with the meat mixture. Combine the beans, the tomatillos, and ½ cup water in the skillet used for the meat. Simmer gently until heated through, about 10 minutes; add salt and pepper to taste. Pour the tomatillo mixture over the meat layer in the pan. Cover with aluminum foil and bake for 20 minutes.

Uncover and sprinkle with the cheese. Return to oven and bake, uncovered, until the cheese melts. Serve with sour cream and salsa as toppings.

NOTE: Tomatillos are related to tomatoes but are tart even when ripe and pale golden. They are usually used while fairly green and firm. To prepare them, peel off the papery husk and then thoroughly rinse the tomatillos to remove the sticky or waxy coating before chopping.

A Farm Story

Here's the story of Brookfield Farm, one of the longest-running and largest CSAs in the United States. In 1976, Claire and David Fortier purchased sixty-four acres of agricultural and forest land. They built a small pole barn, plowed the first fields, and set up Fortier Farm, Inc. In 1980, they started small organic gardens, purchased a cow, and drew up equipment priorities. The farm began selling produce to local wholesalers, and its name was changed to Brookfield Farm.

In 1986, Brookfield Farm became the third CSA in the United States. Fifty-five member households joined in supporting the farm and receiving their share from approximately four acres of vegetable production. Also that year, the first apprentices were hired.

In 1987, the Biodynamic Farmland Conservation Trust, Inc., was created to take on the responsibility of running (owning) the farm and clarifying and expanding the mission to include education of farmers and the public.

By 1991, the CSA had grown to one hundred households. Members paid their share of the running costs and were allowed to take as much of the available produce—from approximately seven acres of vegetable production—as they needed. The apprenticeship program was, by then, taking on two or three trainees each year.

The years from 1992 to 1994 were difficult. The farm struggled to retain members and experienced a financial crisis. (The original founders had passed away, and the original farmers left the farm). The apprenticeship program was eliminated.

In 1995, Dan Kaplan became farm manager. Share structure was changed to reflect changes in local markets, and membership grew to more than five hundred households. Infrastructure, finances, and the membership base were improved. There are now twenty-five acres of vegetable production. The apprenticeship program has been rekindled and blossoms, with consistently more applicants than positions.

RATATOUILLE

MAKES 6 SERVINGS

Farmer Dan Kaplan of Brookfield Farm in Amherst, Massachusetts, gave us this recipe that his apprentice Nicole Goode found on a trip to the south of France. Almost all the ingredients can be found on the farm at the same time.

2 tablespoons olive oil
2 medium bell peppers, cubed
1 medium onion, chopped
1 to 2 garlic cloves, finely chopped
3 medium tomatoes, chopped

1 medium eggplant, peeled and cubed
1 medium zucchini or squash, cubed
Chopped fresh parsley, oregano, and
   basil

Heat the oil in a large, heavy skillet over medium heat. Sauté the peppers, onion, and garlic until soft; stir in the tomatoes, eggplant, zucchini, and herbs. Cover and simmer for about 30 minutes. Voilà!

LAYERED EGGPLANT CASSEROLE

MAKES 4 SERVINGS

Joanne Brieff, a member of the Carnegie Hill/Yorkville CSA in Manhattan, says her mother has been cooking this recipe successfully for fifty-five years; when Joanne makes it herself, she uses stone-ground whole wheat flour, which makes it even better. It's a very adaptable recipe; she often adds other vegetables to the mix and adjusts the amount of cheese. Instead of frying the eggplant slices, you can drizzle them with oil and bake them on a cookie sheet for about thirty minutes in a 350°F oven.

2 to 3 tablespoons vegetable oil
1 large egg
2 tablespoons milk
1/4 cup all-purpose flour, plus more if
   needed
1 large eggplant, peeled and cut into
   1/4-inch-thick slices

1 large onion, finely chopped
4 large tomatoes, cut into 1/4-inch-thick
   slices
4 ounces Monterey Jack cheese, grated
1 tablespoon unsalted butter

Preheat the oven to 350°F. Oil a 2-quart casserole. Beat the egg and milk in a bowl and spread the flour on a plate.

Heat 1 tablespoon of the oil in a large skillet. Dip each slice of eggplant into the egg mixture, and then flour on both sides. Place the slices in the skil-

Sandwiches

When you're making ratatouille, make a lot. If you don't eat it all on the first go-round, you'll have some for sandwiches the next day. Just layer the hot or cold vegetables on bread and add slices of cheese (fresh mozzarella works divinely). Leave it open-faced, or add another slice of bread.

Some people prefer the same combination of vegetables—onions, eggplant, peppers, zucchini, tomatoes (with garlic and herbs)—but in larger pieces. If you want to cook vegetables just for sandwiches, cut the vegetables vertically into thin slices and sauté in olive oil until soft.

let in a single layer and fry until golden on both sides. Continue frying the eggplant in batches, adding oil as necessary, until done.

Layer the fried eggplant, the onion, the tomato, and the cheese until they are all used up; the final layer should be eggplant. Sprinkle any remaining flour (or use another 2 tablespoons flour) over the top. Dot with the butter. Place in the oven, uncovered, for about 45 minutes, until bubbling and the eggplant is tender.

ASIAN FRIED VEGETABLES

MAKES 4 SERVINGS

Tanya Furtado, a professional baker and personal chef, moves around a lot. She's lived in Ohio, Huntington Beach, Seattle, San Antonio, New York, and now in Milwaukee, with her husband, Alex, and their two children, Max and Maya—and she's found a CSA in every city. Many of our midsummer CSA shares will include almost everything needed for this recipe.

¼ cup thinly sliced green onions
3 garlic cloves, finely chopped
1 tablespoon finely chopped peeled fresh ginger
1 teaspoon Asian chili sauce
2 tablespoons soy sauce
2 tablespoons light brown sugar
1 tablespoon balsamic vinegar

2 to 3 tablespoons vegetable oil
1 medium Japanese eggplant, peeled and cut into 1-inch pieces
1 medium zucchini, cut into 1-inch pieces
1 medium red or yellow bell pepper, cut into 1-inch pieces
¼ pound small white mushrooms

Combine the green onions, garlic, ginger, and chili sauce in a cup. Combine ¼ cup water with the soy sauce, brown sugar, and balsamic vinegar in another cup; set both aside.

Heat a large, heavy skillet over high heat. Add 2 tablespoons oil and swirl to coat the pan. Reduce the heat to medium. When the oil sizzles, add the green onion mixture. Stir gently for about 30 seconds, adjusting the heat so the ingredients don't burn. Add the eggplant, zucchini, bell pepper, and mushrooms; cook, stirring, until the vegetables begin to brown, about 4 minutes, adding more oil if necessary.

Stir the soy sauce mixture and add to the pan; toss well. Bring the liquid to a simmer, cover the pan, and simmer until most of the liquid is absorbed— 2 to 3 minutes.

Judith Hausman, a freelance culinary journalist with a regular column in the *Journal News* in White Plains, New York, and a member of Chefs Collaborative, sent us this recipe from a CSA family that she had written an article about and found so fascinating that she stayed in contact with them. The 125-acre Ryder Farm near Brewster, New York, is farmed by Hall Gibson, who married into the Ryder family, owners of that acreage since 1795. Most of Gibson's career was spent with the federal government in Washington until he retired early in 1976 to save the family farm. He says, "It's a very dear place. It's one of the few small farms that survives in our area and the only certified organic farm in Westchester and Putnam Counties." In addition to their "pick-your-own raspberries" program, Gibson had participated in New York City's Union Square Market, but gave it up after twenty years, on his seventy-sixth birthday, to create his CSA. This recipe is from Belle Ryder, the ninety-year-old granddaughter-in-law of Stephen Ryder, who started the farm.

BREAD AND BUTTER PICKLES

MAKES ABOUT 8 PINTS

6 pounds unwaxed cucumbers
3 pounds onions, thinly sliced
½ cup kosher or pickling salt
4½ cups sugar

4 cups cider or white wine vinegar
2 tablespoons mustard seeds
1½ tablespoons celery seeds
1 tablespoon ground turmeric

Trim and cut the cucumbers into ¼-inch-thick slices. Combine the cucumber slices and onions in a large bowl. Toss with the salt and cover with ice for 3 to 4 hours, replenishing the ice as necessary.

Combine the sugar, vinegar, mustard seeds, celery seeds, and turmeric in a large pot and boil until the sugar dissolves. Drain and rinse the cucumbers and onions and add them to the hot liquid. Slowly return all of it to a full, rolling boil; remove from heat.

Bring a large pot of water to a boil and sterilize eight 1-pint jars, new lids, and rings. Keep the water simmering. Spoon the hot cucumber mixture into the jars, leaving ½-inch headroom between the liquid and the top of the jar. Add the lids and rings to seal, and process in the hot-water bath for 10 minutes. Remove and set aside to cool. Check the seals, label, and store in a cool, dry place.

PEPERONATA

MAKES 4 SERVINGS

Katherine Kelly, owner of Full Circle Farm in Kansas City, Kansas, grew up outside Wichita. She moved to Minneapolis–Saint Paul and eventually to Boston and Kansas City, doing everything from program development to fund-raising to marketing; on the side, she learned organic farming. Her partner, Carol Burns, who is Teton-Lakota-American, is a documentary filmmaker as well as a farmer. This recipe is from Full Circle member Lee Alexander.

2 tablespoons olive oil
1 large onion, cut into 1-inch pieces, layers separated
1 garlic clove, finely chopped
5 medium bell peppers, thinly sliced

1 1/4 cups prepared tomato sauce (see Basic Tomato Sauces, page 30)
Salt and freshly milled black pepper

Heat the oil in a large frying pan over medium heat. Add the onion and garlic; sauté until the onion begins to brown, about 3 minutes. Add the peppers and tomato sauce. Cover and cook until the peppers are just tender, about 8 minutes. Season to taste with salt and pepper and serve.

NUTMEG-WHIPPED SQUASH

MAKES 4 SIDE-DISH SERVINGS

This simple side dish from Marleen Littera is especially good served with ham. She's been a member of Bluebird Hills Farm CSA for five years. To make it even easier, the squash could be roasted whole and the meat scooped out into a bowl to whip with the flavorings.

2 small or 1 large winter squash, peeled and cut into thick slices
2 tablespoons unsalted butter

1 tablespoon light brown sugar
1 teaspoon ground nutmeg
1/2 teaspoon salt

Bring the squash and water to cover by 1 inch to a boil in a large saucepan over high heat. Cover and cook over low heat until the squash is soft, about 20 minutes.

Drain well and add the butter, brown sugar, nutmeg, and salt. Whip with an electric mixer until smooth.

This recipe was submitted by Jon Grommons of Five Springs Farm CSA in Bear Lake, Michigan. Jon and his wife, Jacquelynn, became interested in their local CSA when they were restaurateurs in the area. If you can't get green coriander berries from your CSA, you can substitute 1/4 cup chopped fresh cilantro.

SUMMER KABOBS

MAKES 4 SERVINGS

2/3 cup olive oil

1/3 cup lime juice

4 garlic cloves, finely chopped

1 small hot red pepper, finely chopped

3/4 teaspoon salt

10 green coriander berries

12 small red potatoes

12 small onions, unpeeled

12 cherry or pear tomatoes

4 fennel bulbs, cut into 1-inch pieces

4 jalapeño peppers, cut into 1-inch pieces

3 small zucchini, cut into 1-inch pieces

3 large bell peppers, cut into 1-inch pieces

3 Japanese eggplants, peeled and cut into 1-inch pieces

3 small summer squash, cut into 1-inch pieces

Combine the oil, lime juice, garlic, hot red pepper, salt, and coriander berries in a very large bowl. Set aside.

Boil the potatoes in salted water to cover until just beginning to soften but still quite firm, about 8 minutes. Remove with a slotted spoon to a colander and drain well. Add the onions to the boiling water and cook for 3 minutes. Drain and plunge into ice water. Remove the onion skins, rinse the onions, and add to the potatoes.

Combine the drained potatoes and onions with the tomatoes, fennel, jalapeño peppers, zucchini, bell peppers, eggplant, and squash in the bowl with the oil-and-lime-juice mixture. Toss to coat the vegetables. Cover and refrigerate for 1 to 2 hours.

Preheat a grill. Thread all the vegetables except the tomatoes randomly onto 12 long metal or presoaked bamboo skewers. Thread the tomatoes onto 1 or 2 separate skewers. Grill the mixed vegetables over the hot coals for 10 to 15 minutes, until just tender. Turn and baste with the marinade frequently. Grill the tomatoes for 1 to 2 minutes.

To serve, with tongs, transfer a tomato to the end of each mixed-vegetable skewer.

ZUCCHINI-BRAN BREAD

MAKES 2 (8-INCH) OR
3 (6-INCH) LOAVES

Beth Staggenborg of Boulder Belt CSA in Cincinnati, Ohio, sent us this recipe. She said that she loves zucchini bread but wanted a recipe that wasn't so rich and full of fat, and that, surprisingly, it was difficult to find such an item. Eventually, she discovered the basics of this recipe on the Web and added some ingredients from other zucchini bread recipes and directions from her mother's cranberry bread recipe. It doesn't make a light loaf; it's rather dense, but the flavor is outstanding, the texture is nutty and crunchy, and it freezes well.

3 large eggs
¾ cup vegetable oil
½ cup granulated or raw sugar
¼ cup packed light brown sugar
2 tablespoons honey
2 teaspoons vanilla extract
1 cup all-purpose flour
1 cup whole wheat flour

⅓ cup oat bran cereal
3 tablespoons wheat germ
1 teaspoon baking soda
1 teaspoon ground cinnamon
½ teaspoon salt
2½ cups finely chopped raw zucchini
½ cup chopped nuts
½ cup dark raisins

Preheat the oven to 325°F. Grease two 8-inch or three 6-inch loaf pans.

Beat together the eggs, oil, granulated and brown sugars, honey, and vanilla in a large bowl. Stir together the all-purpose and whole wheat flours, bran cereal, wheat germ, baking soda, cinnamon, and salt in a medium bowl; stir the flour mixture into the egg mixture to make a stiff dough. Fold in the zucchini, nuts, and raisins.

Divide the batter among the baking pans. Bake 8-inch loaves for 40 minutes, 6-inch loaves for 30 minutes. Let cool on a wire rack for at least 15 minutes before slicing.

We like to encourage people to think of making pumpkin pie all year round. Pumpkin freezes beautifully and there is no reason why it should be a fall-only treat.

PUMPKIN PIE

Pastry for 1 (9-inch) single-crust pie
   (see page 21)
2 cups pumpkin puree
3 large eggs
1/4 cup packed light brown sugar
1 1/2 teaspoons ground cinnamon

1 teaspoon ground ginger
1/2 teaspoon ground nutmeg
1/2 teaspoon salt
1/4 teaspoon ground allspice
1/4 teaspoon ground cloves
1 1/2 cups half-and-half

Preheat the oven to 450°F. Prepare the piecrust. On a floured board, roll out the pastry to make an 11-inch round; fit into a standard 9-inch pie pan. Fold over the edges of the dough and flute. Pierce the dough all over with a fork, then press a piece of heavy-duty aluminum foil directly into the pie shell. Bake for 6 minutes, remove the foil, and bake for about 4 more minutes, or until the shell is just beginning to brown. Remove from the oven and set aside.

Beat together the pumpkin puree, eggs, brown sugar, cinnamon, ginger, nutmeg, salt, allspice, and cloves in a large bowl. Gradually beat in the half-and-half until the mixture is smooth.

Pour into the pie shell and bake for 10 minutes. Reduce the heat to 300°F and continue baking for 30 to 40 minutes, until the filling is almost set. A sharp knife inserted slightly off center will come out almost clean. The center of the pie should not be completely firm. Let cool to room temperature and serve with whipped cream. Store any leftovers in the refrigerator.

BUTTERNUT–APPLE CRISP BARS

MAKES 9 SERVINGS

Squash and apples are a natural combination; you just don't usually see them together in desserts. These spicy bars are a great way to pair these two items from your autumn CSA shares. This recipe comes from Mountain Harvest Organics in Hot Springs, North Carolina.

3 cups sliced peeled butternut squash
3 cups sliced peeled tart apples
1 cup packed light brown sugar
2 teaspoons lemon juice
1 teaspoon ground cinnamon
1/8 teaspoon ground cloves

1 cup all-purpose flour
1/2 teaspoon salt
6 tablespoons unsalted butter, softened
1/3 cup chopped nuts
Ice cream (optional)

Preheat the oven to 350°F. Grease a 9-inch square baking pan.

Combine the squash and apple slices with 1/2 cup of the brown sugar, the lemon juice, the cinnamon, and the cloves, tossing gently, in a large bowl. Turn into the prepared pan, cover with aluminum foil, and bake for 30 minutes.

Meanwhile, combine the flour, the remaining 1/2 cup brown sugar, and the salt. Stir in the butter with a fork until crumbly. Add the nuts. Spread evenly over the squash-apple mixture. Bake uncovered for 40 minutes more. Cut into 9 squares; top with ice cream, if desired, and serve.

CHAPTER NINE

ROOTS AND TUBERS

Roots and tubers are the underground storehouses where plants conserve their food and water. High in energy-providing carbohydrates, they are a staple item in our national diet as well as in our CSA shares. Each week, we have a selection of roots and tubers and watch these versatile and easy-to-store vegetables grow from babies in June to winter "keepers" in the late fall. And, whether we get beets, carrots, Jerusalem artichokes, parsnips, potatoes, radishes, rutabagas, sweet potatoes, turnips, or the occasional specialties, someone at the CSA site will have a wonderful new recipe for us all to try. In the past, because roots and tubers were usually not difficult to grow, produced abundantly, and stored well, they were considered food staples of the poor. Today, however, they may be found starring on the fall and winter menus of the most upscale restaurants.

Of the roots and tubers we get in our CSA shares, beets, carrots, celeriac, parsnips, radishes, and turnips originated in the Eastern Hemisphere, and Jerusalem artichokes, potatoes, and sweet potatoes originated in the West.

Beets developed from an aquatic plant that had been growing around the Mediterranean since well before classical authors mentioned their cultivation. The red beet is sometimes called the Roman beet, but golden beets were growing in the same area at the same time. However, it was not until the sixteenth century that beets were bred to have a round and meaty root rather than a long, thin one.

Carrots originated in western Asia and Europe and were thin and deep red until after the sixteenth century. At about that time, they were brought to the Americas and were said to be well received by the native inhabitants because of their sweetness and color.

Celeriac has appeared in botanical and culinary writings since the sixteenth century. Also called celery root, it was quite popular in Europe, where it was easier to grow and store than celery. Except for *céleri rémoulade,* which has continued to be a "regular" at French restaurants, celeriac was pretty much ignored in North America. Recently, chefs have rediscovered this crunchy, mild-flavored root and are using it in new and creative ways.

Parsnips had an origin that paralleled that of the carrot and were often considered a type of carrot. Despite their unique flavor, in medieval times, parsnips were a popular food because of their sweetness and because they made a satisfying, high-carbohydrate meal. By the eighteenth century, parsnips had fallen from favor as more intense sources of sweetness had become available and mild-flavored, high-carbohydrate roots and tubers had arrived from the Americas.

Radishes probably originated in western Asia, and several varieties were in use during classical times. They were taken to North America by early colonists and raised for use in salads and relishes. As they were adapted to different climates, preferences, and uses, many variations in size, shape, and "bite" developed.

Turnips were one of the earliest European vegetables to be cultivated. They were carried to China in classical times and are still used in some form in most of the world's cuisines.

Rutabagas are a variety of turnip that is large and has pale golden flesh. They are associated with the Scandinavian countries but are available in North America as well.

Jerusalem artichokes are not related to artichokes and have nothing to do with Jerusalem. They are a North American relative of the sunflower, and it is thought that their inaccurate name comes from a corruption of "*girasole,*" the Italian word for sunflower and from the fact that, when cooked, they taste a bit like an artichoke. They were taken to Europe very early in the seventeenth century, where they made quite a hit because of their sweetness, but interest faded and they have only recently been easily available in markets in both Europe and America.

Potatoes are native to South America and were carried to Europe by early explorers in the sixteenth century. They were not immediately accepted because, since they were members of the nightshade family, it was rumored that they were poisonous. It took several centuries of persuasion for them to become the staple vegetable of northern Europe, and potatoes came to North America with European colonists at the same time.

Sweet potatoes are also of South American origin and were one of many roots and tubers that Columbus and his crew tasted in 1492. They were taken back to Europe and were very popular because of their sweetness. Although North Americans sometimes confuse the two, sweet potatoes are not yams. Yams are large tubers of the genus *Dioscorea* that are native to Southeast Asia, Africa, and South America. They are rarely grown in North America and have even been displaced by the sweet potato in some of their places of origin.

Roots and tubers are planted in several different ways. Some, such as beets, carrots, and turnips, grow from seeds, and others, such as sweet potatoes, grow from sprouts that come from seed potatoes, while potatoes are raised from chunks of mature potato that contain one or more "eyes." Most roots and tubers like cool, moist weather and flourish in northern climates. In fact, parsnips can be left in the ground over the winter and harvested as needed. They actually seem to get sweeter after a good frost. Sweet potatoes, however, prefer the heat and are grown mostly in our southern states.

Roots and tubers are best when freshly harvested because they dry out and eventually shrivel when stored indoors in a warm, dry location. Look for smooth, firm, well-shaped, medium-sized, intensely colored vegetables that are not wrinkled, flabby, dry-looking, or cracked. If possible, it is best to avoid gnarled ones because they are harder to peel and you are likely to lose more vegetable by the time you get the skin off. Buy carrots and beets with tops when you can because the freshness and quality of the tops give you a clue as to how long they have been out of the ground.

After You Pick Up or Buy

If you have followed our advice above and brought home carrots or beets with the tops, remove the tops before storing the vegetables. Discard the carrot tops; the beet tops will make delicious cooked greens (see chapter 3). Carrots, beets, Jerusalem artichokes, and turnips store best, unwashed, in perforated vegetable bags in the refrigerator. Under these conditions, they should maintain their quality for two to three weeks. Potatoes and sweet potatoes are best when stored in a cool, moist place out of the refrigerator. Do not store potatoes with onions; it is not good for either one of them.

Preparing Uncooked

Beets, carrots, celeriac, Jerusalem artichokes, and turnips can be served un-cooked. While if young and tender enough, all but celeriac could be scrubbed and not peeled, peeling definitely makes them more palatable. Once peeled, they can be sliced, cut into cubes, or shredded and used as crudités, in salads or relishes, and as garnishes.

Preparing Cooked

BLANCHING is a great way to reduce the roasting or grilling time necessary for roots and tubers, so they can be mixed with quicker-cooking items in vegetable mixtures, kabobs, or stir-fries. Give them a little longer than most vegetables, say, 5 to 7 minutes.

BOILING is a fast, low-fat way to tenderize roots and tubers. Whether whole or sliced, they should be cooked until crisp-tender, as they will hold the heat and continue to cook after they have been removed from the cooking liquid. Beets can be boiled in their skin until just tender and then peeled, making the peeling very easy.

BRAISING is frequently chosen for cooking root vegetables. Whether done in the oven or on top of the stove, the long, low-temperature cooking brings out their sweetness, and the use of stock or wine for the cooking liquid and of herbs or spices for the seasoning adds flavor to the mild-flavored vegetables.

Root-Cellaring

If you have any spot in your house to set aside for a root cellar, this old-fashioned storage technique can double the storage life of roots and tubers. What you need is an area with higher than usual humidity in which you can maintain a temperature between 32° and 40°F. A basement area with a dirt floor, the sheltered stairs to an outdoor basement entryway, or a sheltered basement window well can often meet those requirements. Securely cover the containers so that visitors can't get in but air can still circulate in and out. For long-term storage in a root cellar, layer vegetables in sand in shallow boxes.

DEEP-FRYING Although any root or tuber can be deep-fried, potatoes are without question at the top of the list for actual preparation. While they are not often prepared at home, French fries have been elevated to an art form in restaurants in many parts of Europe and the United States. Sweet potato fries are now available in many restaurants as well.

GLAZING is as popular with baby roots and tubers as it is with baby onions. Once they have been boiled to crisp-tender separately, they are often combined for the glazing process. Just drain off most of the cooking liquid, add 1 tablespoon sugar, 1 tablespoon unsalted butter, and freshly milled black pepper to taste. Cook them, uncovered, over low heat until only a few tablespoons of the syrup produced remain. Stir or shake the pan so the vegetables are coated in the syrup and start to brown slightly.

ROASTING concentrates the sweetness and mellows the flavors of roots and tubers. Peel the vegetables and cut them into 1-inch chunks if they are larger than that. Toss them in a little oil; add salt and freshly milled black pepper to taste and any of the sturdier herbs such as thyme or rosemary. Spread each kind of vegetable out in a separate pan or tray and roast them at 400°F until they are crisp-tender, 20 to 45 minutes depending upon size, type of vegetable, and age. Stir them occasionally and check for doneness every 10 to 12 minutes.

With the exception of beets and carrots, roots and tubers are best stored in a root cellar if you can find any space that meets the requirements (see page 187). Beets and carrots can both be canned or pickled, and carrots can be frozen successfully. Because of their high moisture content, other roots and tubers lose their texture and become mushy or grainy when frozen.

Root and Tuber Nutrition

Roots and tubers are high in carbohydrates, contain moderate to high amounts of dietary fiber, and are especially rich in potassium. Despite their high sugar and starch content, they are remarkably low in calories if not cooked or served with high-calorie ingredients. Carrots and sweet potatoes are very high in beta-carotene, which has recently been found to reduce the risk of various cancers. Potatoes, sweet potatoes, and parsnips contain vitamin C, and potatoes, parsnips, and Jerusalem artichokes are high in the B vitamins. As for minerals, in addition to potassium, beets and Jerusalem artichokes are high in iron, and parsnips are high in phosphorus.

MASHED POTATO PANCAKES (CHREMSLACH)

MAKES 48 PANCAKES

A great way to use up leftover mashed potatoes! If you're using leftover potatoes, bring them to room temperature and mash them again, or put them through a ricer or food mill before combining with the eggs.

2 pounds potatoes, peeled and cut into chunks
2 large eggs

Salt and freshly milled black pepper
Oil

Cook the potatoes in boiling salted water until tender, about 20 minutes. Drain well and mash, or, even better, put them through a ricer.

Separate the eggs; place the whites in a large bowl and the yolks in a cup. Beat the egg whites with an electric mixer until stiff peaks form.

Beat the yolks with a fork and gently fold them into the whites. Add the potatoes, a few tablespoons at a time, and stir gently after each addition to combine. Add salt and pepper to taste.

Heat the oil in a large skillet. Drop tablespoons of the potato-egg batter into the oil and fry until golden, then turn and fry the other side, 1 to 2 minutes per side. Transfer the pancakes to paper towels to drain, then serve.

CREAMY TURNIP SOUP

MAKES 6 SERVINGS

Of all the recipes that Debby Kavakos of Stoneledge Farm in South Cairo, New York (who delivers to our CSA), has given us, this is the most requested. When the ungainly turnips of autumn begin to arrive, members look at them doubtfully and sometimes leave them behind. But everyone who tries this soup becomes a turnip lover. It can be made with water instead of stock, but the stock makes the soup much richer and tastier.

1 tablespoon unsalted butter or
   margarine
1 cup coarsely chopped onions or leeks
4 cups chopped peeled turnips
2 cups chicken or vegetable stock or
   water
2 tablespoons minced fresh parsley

1 tablespoon sugar
1 tablespoon lemon juice
1 bay leaf
1/8 teaspoon freshly milled black
   pepper
1 cup milk
1/8 to 1 teaspoon salt

Melt the butter in a Dutch oven over low heat. Add the onions and cook, stirring occasionally, until tender, about 8 minutes. Stir the turnips into the onions, then add the stock, parsley, sugar, lemon juice, bay leaf, and pepper. Cover and simmer for 45 minutes, or until the turnips are very tender.

Remove the bay leaf and puree the turnip mixture in a blender or food processor. Return the puree to the pan; add the milk and salt to taste (if you used salted stock, you will need less salt). Heat the soup just to a boil; divide into 6 warm soup bowls and serve.

ROASTED-POTATO SOUP

Molly Petersons of Molly's Island Garden in Langley, Washington, has found that a splash of unexpected color on traditional vegetables wakes up the appetite. So, her fields are teeming with at least fifteen types of purple vegetables—ranging from purple string beans to purple potatoes to purple cauliflower. Member Shirley Jantz uses all kinds of potatoes in this soup and finds that the ones that can be sliced the most thinly—like organic golden russets—make the crispiest garnishes.

4 medium russet potatoes, peeled, thinly sliced, and cut into small squares

4 garlic cloves, sliced

1 to 2 tablespoons toasted sesame oil or olive oil

1 teaspoon salt

1 teaspoon freshly milled black pepper

2 to 3 cups vegetable stock or salted water

1 cup plain soy or rice milk (or cow's milk, if you prefer)

1/2 cup half-and-half (optional)

1 tablespoon garlic powder

1 tablespoon Italian seasoning

1 teaspoon ground cumin

1 teaspoon ground nutmeg

1 teaspoon ground red pepper

Grated Parmesan cheese (optional)

Chopped fresh flat-leaf parsley (optional)

Chopped fresh or dried thyme (optional)

Cracked black peppercorns (optional)

Preheat the oven to 400°F. Place half of the potatoes and garlic in a 13- by 9-inch baking pan; add the sesame oil. Turn the potatoes and garlic to coat with the oil, sprinkle with 1/2 teaspoon of the salt and 1/2 teaspoon of the pepper. Roast for 15 to 20 minutes, until crispy on one side; turn and roast for another 15 to 20 minutes, until the potatoes are tender.

Meanwhile, bring the stock to a boil in a large saucepan and add the remaining potatoes and garlic. Simmer until tender, about 10 minutes. Puree the mixture in a blender, leaving it as thick as possible. You may need to puree in batches, depending on the size of the blender.

Return the mixture to the pan, add the soy milk and half-and-half, if using, as needed for creaminess and to thin to the desired consistency. Add the garlic powder, Italian seasoning, cumin, nutmeg, red pepper, and remaining 1/2 teaspoon salt and 1/2 teaspoon pepper.

When the roasted potatoes are done, add to the soup base. Divide among 6 bowls and top with Parmesan cheese, parsley, thyme, and cracked black peppercorns, if desired, and serve.

BEET AND APPLE SLAW

MAKES 10 SIDE-DISH SERVINGS

Chefs Christine Wansleben and Valeria Flynn of A Sharper Palate Catering Company in Richmond, Virginia, gave us this easy recipe. They recommend it as a "fantastic recipe for the summer" and told us that when they serve it, all of the main ingredients are purchased at the local growers' market. Their company is an enthusiastic supporter of local agriculture and hosts many events for Virginia agribusiness throughout the year.

1 pound beets, peeled and grated
1 pound Granny Smith apples,
  peeled and grated
½ pound Savoy cabbage, very thinly
  sliced

Salt and freshly milled black pepper
¾ cup sugar
¾ cup cider vinegar
¾ cup prepared mayonnaise

Combine the beets, apples, and cabbage in a large nonreactive bowl. Season with salt and pepper to taste and set aside.

Combine the sugar and vinegar in a small saucepan. Warm over very low heat, stirring, until the sugar is dissolved. Set aside until completely cool. Very gradually whisk the mixture into the mayonnaise in a small bowl. Add more salt and pepper to taste.

Fold the dressing into the slaw mixture; cover and refrigerate for about 3 hours. Stir again before serving.

GVOCSA and Elizabeth Henderson

The Genesee Valley Organic Community Supported Agriculture group (GVOCSA) began as a project of Politics of Food with twenty-six members in 1989, and has expanded yearly. Farmers Elizabeth Henderson, Greg Palmer, and Ammie Chickering grow the food at Peacework Organic Produce at Crowfield Farm, near Newark, New York (which supplies the vegetables, herbs, and flowers for the GVOCSA). Elizabeth Henderson is among the most ardent and articulate supporters of CSA. She is the co-author (with Robyn Van En) of *Sharing the Harvest: A Guide to Community-Supported Agriculture*, the inspirational yet highly practical handbook of the CSA movement. In 1999, she said this when accepting the "Spirit of Organic" Award at the Natural Foods Expo: "Organic farming is Peacework—part of the striving for peace among humans and between humans and all the other creatures of the earth above- and belowground. My hope for the future is that the industry that has formed around organic agriculture will remain true to the "Spirit of the Organ," and serve as a model of a food system in which fair and equitable trading and community relations assure a place for small farms and local businesses in a world of peace and abundance."

POTATO LASAGNA WITH PESTO SAUCE

MAKES 6 SERVINGS

Just a few weeks after arriving from Italy to work with one of the families in the Carnegie Hill/Yorkville CSA in Manhattan, Fabiana Rigamonti brought this dish to a potluck. It was a big success and everyone wanted the recipe. Soon families all over New York's East Side had a delicious new way to use their organic potatoes and green beans.

4 russet potatoes, peeled or scrubbed
½ pound fresh green beans
3 cups milk
6 tablespoons all-purpose flour
6 tablespoons (¾ stick) unsalted butter
¾ teaspoon salt

¼ teaspoon freshly milled black pepper
1 cup pesto sauce (prepared or homemade)
1 cup grated grana Padano cheese
⅛ teaspoon ground nutmeg (optional)
1 (8-ounce) package no-cook lasagna noodles

Halve and steam or boil the potatoes until almost tender, about 10 minutes. Add the beans and cook until crisp-tender, about 5 minutes more. Drain, reserving 1 cup of the vegetable cooking liquid. Set the potatoes and beans aside until cool enough to handle. Meanwhile, make the white sauce: Stir the milk into the flour in a 1½-quart saucepan; add the butter, salt, and pepper; cook over medium heat, stirring frequently, until thickened.

Heat the oven to 350°F. Lightly butter a 13- by 9-inch baking dish. Cut the potatoes and beans into ⅜-inch pieces and place in a large bowl. Fold in half of the white sauce, the pesto sauce, ¼ cup of the cheese, and the nutmeg, if using.

Place one-third of the pasta (it doesn't have to cover the bottom of the pan) in the buttered baking dish; drizzle with ⅓ cup of the vegetable cooking liquid. Add half of the vegetable mixture, another layer of pasta, the remaining vegetable mixture, and the remaining pasta.

Drizzle the remaining ⅔ cup vegetable cooking liquid over the top. Spread the remaining white sauce over the top and sprinkle with the remaining ¾ cup cheese. Cover tightly with a sheet of oiled aluminum foil.

Bake the lasagna for 35 minutes; remove the foil and bake for 20 to 25 minutes more, until the mixture bubbles and the top is lightly browned. Cut into 6 servings and, as Fabiana added to the end of her recipe, "Enjoy Your Meal!!!!!"

Meet the Farmer

Sunrise Acres Farm, Cumberland, Maine

Sally Merrill has long cherished her time at Sunrise Acres. As a child growing up in nearby Portland, Maine, she would look forward to her weekend visits to her grandparents who lived on the farm. "I was always connected to the wide-open spaces," Sally says.

But becoming a farmer wasn't part of her plan. Sally, an academic by profession, previously taught political science at Indiana University. But when she returned to the farm to take care of her ailing parents, who had moved out there, she was seduced by the landscape. She has remained there ever since.

In 1983, Sally inherited Sunrise Acres, a 148-acre swath of land so-named because a good portion of it sits on a hill that is often bathed in sunlight. Sally had long admired the concept of Community Supported Agriculture, which she first learned about while living in Japan in the mid-1970s. But the farm didn't become a CSA until 2000.

Sunrise Acres launched its certified organic CSA in 2000. The vegetables are grown on about five acres of her land. (Yes, the shareholders do get some fresh eggs, but it's mostly about veggies.) Sally is passionate about the CSA's role in getting healthy, nutrient-dense food to the local community. She also continues in a kind of teaching role by writing the weekly newsletter, which strives to help members make use of the produce.

The state of Maine, which boasts sandy soil, is potato country. So it's no surprise that Sunrise Acres grows four or five varieties of potatoes, all of which Sally likes to watch flower. The biggest challenge to growing the tubers is the bugs. Oh, and it also takes some time to dig the potatoes up.

But Sally doesn't have a favorite vegetable. They're just all so good. "Each one, as it comes into season, is just so sweet and crisp," she says. She has begun to grow more traditional vegetables after finding that's what members like best. "I had 'Chioggia' beets, for example, beautiful beets with alternating red and white concentric circles, but they didn't go over too well," she recalls. "I just want to promote the idea of eating local organic fresh farm produce, and if people want conventional kinds of vegetables, I'll stick with conventional."

Although Sally herself inherited a family farm, she does not think preserving farm lineages is that important. "What is important is that farms are passed on to the next generation, genetically or not, that is committed to stewardship," Sally says. "Bloodline is a secondary matter."

This recipe was created by Alison Clarke, a member of New York's Genesee Valley Organic CSA, one of the first CSA farms in the Northeast. Beet burgers were a hit at a 1993 Organically Grown Week dinner and kept guests happy even when the speaker was over an hour late. After you've made them once, experiment with different amounts of garlic, parsley, and red pepper. Genesee Valley members are garlic lovers and add garlic liberally.

BEET BURGERS

MAKES 6 BURGERS

2 cups grated peeled beets
   (about 12 ounces)
2 cups grated peeled carrots
   (about 6 ounces)
1 cup cooked brown rice
1 cup grated Cheddar cheese
1 cup sunflower seeds, toasted
2 large eggs, beaten

½ cup sesame seeds, toasted
½ cup grated onion (about 1 medium)
¼ cup vegetable oil
3 tablespoons all-purpose flour
3 tablespoons chopped fresh parsley
2 to 4 garlic cloves, finely chopped
2 tablespoons soy sauce
Ground red pepper

Preheat the oven to 350°F. Generously grease a rimmed baking sheet.

Combine all ingredients in a large bowl.

Form the mixture into patties and bake for 25 to 30 minutes, until firm and the vegetables are cooked through.

Taste Over Yield

That's the motto at Live Earth Farm, a twenty-acre family farm in the foothills of the Santa Cruz Mountains, near Watsonville, California, run by Tom and Constance Broz and their son David. They say, "Great taste comes from selecting the right crop varieties, and harvesting at the optimum stage of ripeness. For example, our strawberries, which we promise you will get addicted to, are picked fully ripe only hours before you pop them into your mouth. Our tomatoes are dry-farmed and have a flavor so sweet and intense, you'll never forget them." At Live Earth, great taste is achieved by growing many different varieties of the same type of crop and selecting the most flavorful ones. The farm is 100 percent organic and goes beyond what the law requires to grow food that is vibrant and alive, nurturing their soil with homemade compost, cover crops, and crop rotation. Tom Broz, who grew up in Ecuador, sells his crops through his CSA and at a farmers' markets. "It's a perfect combination for ensuring that I can grow and sell the right way," he says.

SPINACH GNOCCHI

MAKES 8 SERVINGS

Debbie Palmer, a member of Live Earth Farm CSA in Watsonville, California, contributed this traditional recipe. When spinach is in season, it is a good idea to double the recipe and freeze some for later in the year. Debbie prefers waxy, creamy potatoes like fingerlings or Yukon Gold, but if she has only starchier types like russets or Peruvian purples, she doesn't let that stop her. She doesn't peel her potatoes—she loves little bits of potato skin in her gnocchi. She also says this recipe is equally good made with chard or even beet greens, if you don't have spinach.

½ pound potatoes
Salt
1 large bunch spinach

2 egg yolks
1 tablespoon olive oil
1¾ to 2 cups all-purpose flour

Peel or just scrub potatoes, cut into pieces and boil in salted water until tender (15 to 20 minutes). Drain, allow to cool (so that the egg yolk doesn't cook when added), then mash well (don't use a food processor).

Wash spinach, remove tough stems, and steam over boiling water a minute to two, just until wilted. Drain, and when cool enough to handle, squeeze as much water from the spinach as you can. Place the spinach on a cutting board and chop it well. Mix the spinach into the mashed potatoes. Add egg yolks and salt, and mix well.

Work in about ¾ to 1 cup of the flour, kneading into a dough. Add additional flour to make a firm, smooth dough that does not stick to your fingers.

Divide dough into tennis-ball-sized pieces. On a floured surface, roll each piece into a rope about ½ inch in diameter. Cut into 1-inch segments. With floured hands, round up the segments into little egg shapes, then roll them under the tines of a fork (also dipped in flour) to create ridges.

If you want to freeze the gnocchi, place them on wax paper on a cookie sheet (close but not touching) and freeze. Remove from sheets, then store in zippered plastic bags in freezer.

To cook, drop the gnocchi into a large pot of boiling salted water (do not crowd them). Whether you are cooking frozen or freshly made gnocchi, they are ready when they rise to the surface. Remove with a slotted spoon. Serve with your favorite sauce or with melted butter, minced parsley, and Parmigiano-Reggiano.

SPAETZLE WITH ROOT VEGETABLES

MAKES 6 SERVINGS

Shelley Boris is executive chef of Bill Brown's Restaurant and Bar in Garrison, New York, a town about fifty miles north of New York City in the scenic and socially conscious Hudson Valley highlands. Shelley seeks out local fruits and vegetables to serve in her restaurant because she prizes their superior taste and believes in sustainable agriculture. "I want to have farmers and good safe land everywhere," says Shelley, who gets some of her produce from Four Winds Farms, a CSA in nearby Gardiner. Shelley is fond of this spaetzle recipe because it showcases underappreciated root vegetables, and the homespun noodles somehow make parsnips and turnips less intimidating.

1 1/3 cups milk
8 large eggs plus 4 large yolks
Salt
1/4 teaspoon freshly milled black
    pepper
1/8 teaspoon freshly grated nutmeg
4 1/4 cups all-purpose flour
Chopped fresh parsley and chives

3 to 4 cups mixed root vegetables,
    such as parsnips, turnips, carrots,
    sweet potatoes, and winter squash
1/4 cup extra-virgin olive oil
2 tablespoons unsalted butter
1 1/2 cups unseasoned dried bread
    crumbs

Several hours before preparing, whisk together the milk, eggs, egg yolks, 2 teaspoons salt, the pepper, and nutmeg in a large bowl. Sift the flour over the mixture and whisk in until smooth. Stir in the herbs. Cover and refrigerate for at least 1 hour or until ready to cook.

One hour before serving, preheat the oven to 400°F. Toss the mixed vegetables with the oil and 1/2 teaspoon salt and roast for 45 to 55 minutes, until tender and slightly browned.

Bring 3 quarts salted water to a boil in a large sauce pot. In several batches, pour the batter into a spaetzle maker or colander that sits securely on the sauce pot and press the spaetzle into the boiling water. Boil until the spaetzle rise to the top, about 1 minute. With a slotted spoon, transfer the spaetzle to a bowl of ice water. Repeat until all the batter has been boiled.

To serve, melt the butter in a large skillet; add the bread crumbs and sauté for 3 minutes. Drain the spaetzle very well and add to the crumbs along with the vegetables; toss to combine. Divide among 6 serving plates and serve with a salad.

What's the difference between buying straight from a farmer and buying from a supermarket? Shari Sirkin of Dancin' Roots Farm in Portland, Oregon, says that her CSA members "can look me in the eye and know that the food I'm giving them is fresh and healthy." This recipe is her way of using winter vegetables, and she encourages us to vary the ingredients (sometimes she makes it with just one or two root vegetables). She makes a whole roaster-pan full during busy fall weekends, then just scoops out what she needs and reheats it every night.

ROASTED ROOTS WITH WINTER GREENS

MAKES 8 SERVINGS

2 pounds potatoes, peeled and cut into large pieces

6 medium carrots, peeled and cut into large pieces

4 medium parsnips, peeled and cut into large pieces

4 medium rutabagas, peeled and cut into large pieces

4 medium turnips, peeled and cut into large pieces

Olive oil

3 medium beets, peeled and cut into large pieces

Salt and freshly milled black pepper

1 tablespoon chopped fresh herb, such as rosemary, summer savory, thyme, or a mixture

1 large onion, chopped

4 cups thickly sliced collards, kale, Swiss chard, bok choy, spinach, or arugula

1 ½ to 2 cups crumbled feta cheese

Preheat the oven to 425°F. Combine the potatoes, carrots, parsnips, rutabagas, and turnips in one or two large roasting pans; toss them with the oil to coat lightly. In a separate pan, toss the beets with a little oil. Add salt and pepper to taste and your choice of herbs to all the vegetables. Roast for about 1 hour, or until the roots are tender.

When the roots are just about done, heat 1 tablespoon oil in a large skillet over medium heat. Add the onion and sauté until it is soft. Add the greens and ¼ cup water; cook, covered, stirring frequently, until the greens are just tender and still bright green, 3 to 5 minutes.

To serve, place a large scoop of roasted roots on an individual plate; top with a large helping of greens and 3 to 4 tablespoons crumbled feta cheese.

GOLDEN BEET RISOTTO

MAKES 8 SERVINGS

Chef Lou Rook of Annie Gunn's restaurant in Chesterfield, Missouri, makes this elegant dish with locally produced St. Isidore Farm golden beets, Ozark Forest Farm shiitake mushrooms, and Goatsbeard Farm goat cheese. Lou's working relationship with St. Isidore Farm's Bob Loper is particularly close. The farm, located about thirty minutes away from the suburban St. Louis restaurant, grows almost exclusively for Annie Gunn's. Lou says the produce is of a much higher quality than similar items he can get shipped in from California. "The difference is night and day," Lou says. "The fresh herbs are just so much more potent, and the beets are sweeter." Lou's risotto recipe allows for flexibility if you can't get your hands on baby beets. Simply slice up regular-sized beets and quarter them if they are large. And use red beets if you don't have access to the golden variety. Just be aware, Lou says, that you'll end up with pink risotto.

Shiitake Mushroom Relish
    (recipe follows)
8 cups chicken or vegetable stock
1/2 cup olive oil
1/4 cup finely chopped shallots
2 cups arborio rice
1/2 pound baby golden or red beets,
    or large beets, quartered

8 tablespoons (1 stick) unsalted butter
    (optional)
1/4 cup chopped fresh chives
1 ounce Parmesan cheese, grated
Salt and freshly cracked black
    peppercorns
4 ounces goat cheese or 2 ounces
    Parmesan cheese

Prepare the Shiitake Mushroom Relish. Bring the stock to a boil over high heat; reduce the heat to low and hold the stock at a simmer.

Heat the oil in a 4-quart sauce pot; add the shallots and sauté until translucent. Add the rice and stir to coat with the oil. Add about 2 cups of the stock and cook, stirring frequently, until all the stock has been absorbed. Repeat, adding about 2 cups stock at a time, until the rice is just tender and all the stock has been incorporated, 20 to 25 minutes.

Meanwhile, blanch and peel the baby beets. When the risotto is ready, stir in the beets, butter, if using, chives, and Parmesan; season to taste with salt and cracked peppercorns. Divide the mixture among 8 warm soup plates; divide the Shiitake Mushroom Relish among the centers of the plates and garnish with crumbled goat cheese or shaved Parmesan.

Mashed Potatoes

Most people don't need a recipe for mashed potatoes; they have a pretty good idea of how they like them, often based on how their mothers made them, and the concept varies greatly from person to person. You just boil up some baking potatoes in salted water until they are very tender, drain them well, and put them through a potato ricer, mash them with a potato masher, or whip them with an electric beater, gradually adding warm milk or cream or some of the cooking liquid and a few chunks of butter until they reach the consistency you want. And the resulting fluffy bowl of America's quintessential comfort food is ready to serve. But should you want to vary the experience, here are some ideas:

- Cook one or more sliced carrots, turnips, or parsnips with the potatoes and mash them together.
- Cook whole baby red and Peruvian blue potatoes in separate small saucepans until tender, quarter them, and fold into the mashed potatoes.
- Simmer a dozen or so sliced garlic cloves in butter until soft and fold into the mashed potatoes just before serving.
- Top the bowl of mashed potatoes with caramelized onions just before serving.
- Fold chopped fresh chives, green onions, fresh dill, fresh thyme, or mixed fresh herbs into the potatoes once they are mashed.
- Fold quartered olives into the potatoes after they have been mashed.

SHIITAKE MUSHROOM RELISH: Clean 1 pound shiitake mushrooms; discard the stems and slice into ¼-inch strips. Sauté the mushrooms and ¼ cup shallots that have been cut into ¼-inch-thick matchsticks in 1 tablespoon olive oil until just tender. Transfer to a small bowl and stir in 1 tablespoon finely chopped fresh chives, ¼ cup white truffle oil, ½ teaspoon kosher salt, and ⅛ teaspoon cracked black peppercorns.

MARINATED
BEETS

MAKES 4 SERVINGS

Sweetwater Organic Community Farm, located in Tampa, Florida, was founded in 1995 on six acres of suburban property along Sweetwater Creek. Members are encouraged to join in the farmwork. A recent newsletter asked for volunteers this way: "Although the farm's vegetables are some of the most cooperative seedlings around, they still can't be cajoled into planting themselves. If you joined the farm intending to get involved, now is the time! Being there for the start of the season, and following through to the harvest, is a very rewarding experience." The farm also hosts field trips for local schools.

8 medium beets
2 tablespoons walnut oil
1 tablespoon plus 1 teaspoon fruit
    vinegar (raspberry, pear, or cassis)
3 small garlic cloves, crushed or minced
1/2 teaspoon salt

Freshly milled black pepper
1/2 cup crumbled feta cheese
Toasted walnuts
1/4 cup (packed) coarsely minced fresh
    mint leaves
Extra sprigs of mint for garnish

Preheat oven to 400°F. Wrap the beets in aluminum foil with 1/2 inch of stems slightly exposed. Bake for 45 to 50 minutes. Rinse beets under cold running water and rub off the skins. Trim off the stems. Dry beets on paper towels. Slice them in half lengthwise, and then into very thin half-moons.

Place the beets in a bowl. Add the walnut oil, vinegar, garlic, salt, and pepper and mix well. Cover tightly and refrigerate at least 12 hours (24 is best). Stir beets occasionally. (Option: place all ingredients in a Ziploc bag and tumble when you open the refrigerator during the day.)

Serve cold topped with feta cheese, toasted walnuts, and mint.

Members of Carnegie Hill/Yorkville CSA in Manhattan, stopping by to pick up their shares on their way home after work, often ask, "What can I do with these in a hurry for supper?" If it is a bunch of carrots they are holding, this quick microwave recipe is our favorite suggestion.

½ cup orange juice
8 medium carrots, cut into rounds
¼ cup maple syrup

2 tablespoons unsalted butter
2 tablespoons dark raisins
⅛ teaspoon ground nutmeg (optional)

Microwave the orange juice in a 6-cup microwave-safe dish for 1 minute on high power.

Add the carrots to the orange juice. Stir to coat the carrots with the juice. Cover and microwave for 8 to 9 minutes on high power.

Stir in the maple syrup, butter, raisins, and nutmeg, if using. Microwave, uncovered, for 2 minutes on high power. Stir, check for doneness, cook for another 1 minute on high power, if needed.

MICROWAVE MAPLE-GLAZED CARROTS

MAKES 8 SERVINGS

ROSY RADISHES

MAKES 4 SERVINGS

Many people use radishes raw for years and never think of cooking them. But once you give it a try and discover the mild turniplike flavor and pretty pink sauce that results, you will want to serve them this way often.

24 to 28 red radishes (3 to 4 bunches)
¼ teaspoon salt
⅛ teaspoon freshly milled black
  pepper

2 tablespoons unsalted butter
1 small onion, finely chopped
2 tablespoons all-purpose flour
1 tablespoon chopped fresh parsley

Bring 1¾ cups water to a boil in a medium saucepan over high heat; add the radishes, salt, and pepper. Reduce the heat to low and simmer, covered, until the radishes are just tender, 8 to 10 minutes. Drain, reserving the cooking liquid, and set aside.

Meanwhile, melt the butter in a skillet over medium heat. Add the onion and sauté until lightly browned. Whisk in the flour until the onions are uniformly coated. Gradually add the cooking liquid from the radishes, whisking to combine evenly. Simmer, uncovered, for several minutes, until the sauce thickens slightly. Add the radishes and return the mixture to a boil. Taste and add salt and pepper, if necessary. Fold in the parsley and serve.

CHOCOLATE BEET CAKE

MAKES 12 SERVINGS

Letty Flatt, executive pastry chef for Deer Valley Resort in Park City, Utah, and author of *Chocolate Snowball: And Other Fabulous Pastries from Deer Valley Bakery,* created this unusual recipe. She told us that the beets "make the cake moist and sweet—they are the secret ingredient that will never be guessed." Letty met Steve Erickson of Ranui Gardens on a backcountry ski trip, years before he and his wife, Jenny, started farming. She knew about Community Supported Agriculture and signed up right away when the Ericksons started a program, and soon began writing recipes for the CSA.

4 (1-ounce) squares unsweetened
  chocolate, cut into small pieces
4 large eggs
2 cups packed light brown sugar
1/2 cup canola oil
1 teaspoon vanilla extract
2 cups unbleached all-purpose flour

1 1/2 teaspoons baking powder
1 teaspoon baking soda
1/2 teaspoon salt
1 pound red beets, peeled and grated
About 1 3/4 cups cream cheese frosting
  or fudgy chocolate frosting

Preheat the oven to 350°F. Grease two 9-inch round cake pans; line the bottoms with circles of parchment or wax paper and grease the parchment.

Melt the chocolate in the top of a double boiler, over gently boiling water; the upper pan should not touch the water. Keep warm.

Whip the eggs and brown sugar with an electric mixer for about 5 minutes, or until the mixture is noticeably thicker. Add the oil, whipping until it is incorporated. Add the vanilla and melted chocolate and scrape the sides and bottom of the bowl.

Sift together the flour, baking powder, baking soda, and salt. Add to the egg mixture and mix on low speed until well combined, stopping to scrape the bowl. Add the beets and mix well. Pour into the prepared pans. Bake for 40 to 50 minutes, or until the centers spring back when gently pressed. Let cool completely in the pans on wire racks.

With a serrated knife, trim the dome from both cakes so they are flat, not rounded. Trim the sides of the cakes if they seem dry. If you wish, grind the cake trimmings in a food processor or blender and reserve them for garnishing the sides of the cake. Put one of the cake layers on a cardboard circle or a flat serving plate. Spread on 3/4 cup of the frosting. Gently flatten the second cake layer on top. Frost the sides and top of the cake with the remaining 1 cup frosting. If desired, press some of the reserved cake crumbs onto the sides of the cake.

© Letty Flatt

CARROT CAKE

MAKES 12 SERVINGS

Carrots are a favorite crop at Natural Roots Organic Farm in Conway, Massachusetts. Heather Anne Borcy, a member, searched for a carrot cake recipe that was just sweet enough to let the flavor of the carrots dominate.

2 cups all-purpose flour
2 cups sugar
3 teaspoons ground cinnamon
2 teaspoons baking soda
1 teaspoon baking powder
1 teaspoon salt

3 large eggs
1 cup vegetable oil
4 cups grated carrots
1 ½ cups dark raisins
1 ½ cups chopped walnuts
Cream Cheese Frosting (recipe follows)

Preheat the oven to 350°F. Grease two 9-inch round cake pans; line the bottoms of the pans with parchment or wax paper and grease the parchment.

Combine the flour, sugar, cinnamon, baking soda, baking powder, and salt in a large bowl. Beat in the eggs and oil with an electric beater until the mixture is just smooth. Fold in the carrots, the raisins, and 1 cup of the walnuts. Divide the mixture between the two pans.

Bake for 35 to 40 minutes, until the centers spring back when gently pressed. Let cool in the pans on wire racks for 5 minutes. Turn out and let cool completely. Put one of the cake layers on a cardboard circle or a flat serving plate, and spread with frosting. Gently flatten the second layer on top, then frost the sides and top of the cake. with the remaining ½ cup nuts. Store the cake in the refrigerator.

CREAM CHEESE FROSTING: Beat together 1 (8-ounce) package softened cream cheese, 8 tablespoons (1 stick) softened unsalted butter, and 2 teaspoons vanilla extract until smooth. Add 4 cups confectioners' sugar and beat until smooth and fluffy, about 3 minutes.

Eileen Thiel, whose husband, Gene, is known as the potato man at Portland, Oregon, restaurants, gave us this recipe that she had gotten from her mother-in-law. She said that "Gene's mother, Sara, used to make this cake for everyone's birthday, which was often because she had fourteen children." The Thiels were conventional potato farmers in Idaho and moved to Oregon to become organic farmers. Eileen told us that the credit for changing over to organic farming goes to Gene, "because it took so much financial sacrifice and moral fortitude in the face of normal farming practices. He does all the hard work, all the planning and marketing. I am just his sidekick and not a farmer at all. Gene feels that as the American farmer continues farming with chemicals, our land is dying, our food is dying, and we are dying as a nation of an increasingly sick population."

POTATO CAKE

MAKES 12 SERVINGS

2 cups all-purpose flour
2 teaspoons baking powder
4 large eggs
2 cups sugar
½ pound (2 sticks) unsalted butter, softened
1 cup mashed potatoes
1 cup milk
2 tablespoons unsweetened cocoa powder
1 teaspoon ground cinnamon
1 teaspoon ground cloves
1 teaspoon ground nutmeg
1 teaspoon vanilla extract
1 cup dark raisins
1 cup chopped walnuts
Burned sugar frosting or penuche frosting

Preheat the oven to 350°F. Generously grease two 9-inch round cake pans. Sift the flour and baking powder into a small bowl. Separate the eggs, placing the whites in a medium bowl and the yolks in a large bowl. Beat the whites with an electric mixer until stiff but not dry; set aside.

Add the sugar and butter to the bowl with the yolks; beat with the same beaters (no need to rinse) until fluffy. Beat in the mashed potatoes, milk, cocoa, cinnamon, cloves, nutmeg, and vanilla. On low speed, beat in the flour mixture. Fold in the beaten whites, the raisins, and the nuts.

Bake for 25 to 30 minutes, or until the centers spring back when gently pressed. Do not overbake. Let cool for 5 minutes in the pan. Transfer to wire racks and let cool completely, then frost and serve.

CHAPTER TEN

COOKING WITH FRESH HERBS

Herbs are not connected by the way they grow or by family—their common element is distinctive taste. Herbs are used for flavor, not for substance, but those flavors can intensify the most assertive foods and make the blandest ones complex and delicious.

Botanically, the word "herb" has a totally different meaning from its common usage; any plant that does not form a woody stem is herbaceous. Gardeners ignore this definition and grow a wide variety of plants in their herb gardens, including medicinal plants, dye plants, fragrant plants, and plants with historical or religious significance, as well as culinary herbs.

Garlic is among the first flavorings that were cultivated (it was used medicinally as well as in cooking by the Egyptians more than two thousand years ago). The ancient Greek philosophers wrote extensively about the ways herbs affected foods and moods, and the Romans used them in every dish and even carried them into battle. By the Middle Ages, culinary herbs were grown by both the rich and the poor, and herbalists wrote extensive volumes about their use.

In the Field

Most herbs are less demanding than vegetables; many will grow in semi-shade, with little water, in poor, rocky soil (which reminds them of their Mediterranean heritage). And some of our favorite herbs (thyme, oregano, mint) are perennials—once they're established, they'll return year after year. Of course, there are exceptions: Basil needs lots of sun and water; rosemary is frost-tender; parsley is a notoriously finicky germinator. But overall, herbs are easy.

In fact, you might even be able to grow them on your windowsill. If you can provide sunshine and lots of water, a potted herb will live for weeks or even months. Try basil, rosemary, sage, thyme, and oregano and give them plenty of room in their pots. Snip off what you need, never taking more than one-third of the leaves.

Selecting the Best

Fresh herbs should have fresh, crisp-looking leaves that show no signs of dryness or wilting. If you want to use them for cooking, it is best to avoid those that are flowering, because they will have fewer leaves that can go into the dish you are making. However, if you are using the herbs for garnish, flowering ones are a good choice. It is often a good idea to buy fresh herbs that are potted so that they can be used over several weeks and will regenerate as you use them.

After You Pick Up or Buy

Although they're best right after they're harvested—and after you've used fresh-picked basil and other herbs, it's hard to settle for anything else—your herbs will last for about a week if you take a few minutes to care for them. Large bunches, like parsley, dill, basil, and sage, can be placed in a glass (or even a vase) with an inch or two of water at the bottom (don't put in too much water, or the stems will begin to rot). Keep the glass on a counter or upright in the refrigerator. Cut the stems and change the water every few days (does this sound familiar?—it's the same way you store fresh flowers). Smaller sprigs, like thyme, oregano, or rosemary, should be placed in plastic bags or wrapped in damp paper towels and stored in the crisper drawer of the refrigerator.

Preparing

Herbs have so many uses that it's hard to list them all. Here are just a few:

- Mix with soft cheese and use as a dip.
- Chop and sprinkle over baked potatoes or blend into mashed potatoes.

- Sauté briefly in oil or butter, then sauté vegetable, fish, meat, or poultry chunks in the flavored oil.
- Mix into omelets.
- Add to quick-bread batters.
- Mix your favorite fresh herbs with sea salt and rub into meat or fish before broiling or roasting.
- Make herb butter: Chop and mix a few tablespoons of fresh herbs into softened unsalted butter. Put the flavored butter in a mold or form into a log and cover or wrap with wax paper. Serve with bread, corn, potatoes, or pasta, or over vegetables.
- Make herb-flavored croutons: Butter a few slices of thinly sliced bread with herb butter. Cut into cubes and place on a baking sheet. Bake at 300°F until golden. Serve in soups or salads.
- Make herb cream: Heat 1 cup of heavy cream with a little salt and pepper and 1 tablespoon of a very, very finely chopped fresh herb. Use over pasta or vegetables; add Parmesan cheese if desired.

Preserving

Just about all herbs can be preserved; the taste of frozen or dried herbs is not quite as pure as that of fresh, but there's plenty of flavor left.

FREEZING: The easiest way to handle herbs is simply to put them in zippered plastic bags (wash the herbs well and remove the tough ends; whether you chop them or not is up to you). Basil should be blanched for about a minute before it's frozen, or it will turn black; the others don't need it (though their color will be brighter if you do). When they're thawed, they'll be crumbly and should be treated like dry herbs. Or, freeze small portions in ice cube trays and then pop out what you need.

Another way to freeze herbs is to make herb butters (above) or pestos (see pages 212–13). If you're making pesto for the freezer, don't add the cheese until after it's thawed.

DRYING: Preserving herbs by drying them allows you to watch them (and enjoy their perfume) while they are transformed. Simply tie a bunch with a string (or a pretty ribbon) and hang them upside down in a dry spot (keep them away from drafts, cooking fumes, and extreme cold). When they're completely dry, crumble them and store in a glass jar with a tight cover. You'll be surprised at how much more flavorful they are than store-bought dried herbs, which are sometimes two years old by the time you buy them.

If you need to protect your drying herbs from dust or animals, place them in a plastic bag before tying them. They won't be as decorative, but dusty or nibbled herbs aren't very palatable.

MICROWAVING: You can dry herbs in a microwave oven in a matter of seconds; just remember that if you leave them for a second too long, you'll find a pile of ash (or possibly a blazing bouquet). Spread the herbs on a paper towel and cover with another paper towel (dry about a cupful at a time). Microwave on high for 30 seconds; check and repeat for 5 seconds at each try, until the herbs are dry and crumbly. After the first round, don't let it go for more than 5 seconds at a time.

VINEGARS: If you like to use herbs in salad dressings and marinades, you can trap their flavors for later use by placing them in vinegar. Use any clear vinegar (balsamic doesn't work well, but wine vinegars and fruit vinegars are great). Choose a pretty jar with a tight cover or cork and place the herbs—about three to four large sprigs for each cup of vinegar—in it. Cloves of garlic or small chile peppers add taste and ornament. Heat the vinegar to just below boiling, then pour it into the jar. Cover or cork tightly, let cool, and store in a dark, cool place. You may be tempted to display it where the sun hits it, but if you do so, the flavor will fade. If kept under the right conditions, your herb vinegars will be potent for about a year.

Herbs Are Good for You

Although herbs contain vitamins and minerals—parsley is particularly high in vitamins A and C—we usually don't eat enough of them to make a difference. On the other hand, they are low-calorie flavorings that allow us to enjoy vegetables and other foods with much less fat and salt, and in that way contribute to a healthy diet!

ARUGULA "PESTO"

MAKES ¾ CUP

Leslie Markworth, the farmer at Earth Source Organics CSA in Batavia, Ohio, uses this recipe in the spring, well before basil comes into season, when the arugula is booming. She says that it's an excellent way to eat your greens raw; she spreads it on crusty bread, mixes it with noodles, and adds it to sandwiches for a zing. But feel free to enjoy it any way your heart desires.

2 cups loosely packed arugula
¼ cup walnuts
1 to 2 Swiss chard leaves
Green garlic to taste

2 tablespoons Parmesan or Romano
    cheese (optional)
Salt and freshly milled black pepper
¼ cup olive oil

Combine the arugula, walnuts, Swiss chard, garlic, cheese (if using), and salt and pepper to taste in a food processor and process until finely chopped. Gradually add the oil through the feed tube of the processor with the motor running, processing until the mixture is a smooth sauce.

WOOD CREEK HERB FARM PESTO

MAKES ¾ CUP

Brenda Henry of Wood Creek Herb Farm in Rome, New York, submitted the basil pesto recipe she has refined over the years. Brenda grows more than twenty varieties of herbs, and includes them with vegetables in her CSA members' shares. This pesto can be prepared in quantity when the greens are abundant and frozen in 1 tablespoon packages to add to sauces, dips, or cooked vegetables whenever you wish.

⅓ cup pine nuts or walnuts
2 cups loosely packed fresh basil
    leaves, washed and patted dry
½ cup grated Parmesan cheese
3 or 4 large garlic cloves

¼ to ½ teaspoon salt
¼ teaspoon freshly milled black
    pepper
¾ cup olive oil

Preheat the oven to 350°F. Place the pine nuts on a cookie sheet and toast for 8 to 10 minutes, until lightly browned. In a food processor or blender, combine the toasted nuts with the basil, cheese, garlic, salt, and pepper. Process until the ingredients are well chopped.

Salad Dressings

Herbs and salad dressings are perfect partners; you'll find a full dozen salad dressings on pages 54–55, and just about every one of them uses herbs. The base for many salad dressings is oil mixed with a sharp liquid that cuts its oiliness, usually a vinegar or citrus juice. Here are just a few herbal combinations that work with those basic ingredients:

White wine vinegar with rosemary, garlic, and shallots; or fennel, garlic, and parsley
Cider vinegar with dill, garlic, and flower petals
Red wine vinegar with oregano, sage, and garlic
Balsamic vinegar with mustard, thyme, and basil
Lemon juice with thyme and pepper
Orange juice with mint and fennel
Lime juice with cilantro and hot peppers

Gradually drizzle the oil into the mixture through the feed tube or opening in lid with the motor running until mixture reaches the desired consistency. You don't have to add all the oil if the mixture doesn't seem to need it. Refrigerate unused portion and use within 3 days. Discard if allowed to remain unrefrigerated for any length of time.

VARIATION: You can also make this with cilantro instead of basil.

LEMON-BASIL GRILLED CHICKEN

MAKES 4 SERVINGS

At Bluebird Hills Farm, in Springfield, Ohio, Tim and Laurel Shouvlin have added an unusual component to their organic vegetable farm: They raise registered alpacas, whose fleece is sold for fiber. Tim and Laurel consider themselves stewards of the land, and they raise their produce in a manner they feel will best guarantee that their land will improve with each year's use.

½ cup canola oil
¼ cup lemon juice
¼ cup chopped fresh basil,
   or 1 tablespoon dried
2 tablespoons white wine vinegar
2 garlic cloves, finely chopped

1 teaspoon shredded lemon peel
½ teaspoon salt
¼ teaspoon freshly milled black
   pepper
4 boneless, skinless chicken breast
   halves

Combine the oil, lemon juice, half of the basil, the vinegar, garlic, lemon peel, salt, and pepper in a shallow baking dish. Add the chicken breasts and turn to coat on both sides. Refrigerate, covered, for 30 to 45 minutes.

Preheat a charcoal grill or the broiler. Grill or broil the chicken breasts 4 inches from the heat source for about 5 minutes per side, or until the internal temperature reaches 175°F and the chicken is cooked through. Transfer to a clean serving platter and sprinkle with the remaining basil.

QUICK HERB-BROILED SUMMER VEGETABLES

MAKES 4 SERVINGS

Bettina Birch of Flora Bella Farm in central California was the first farmer to submit a recipe for this book. She created this recipe one beastly hot night when her broiler had just been fixed. She served it with a quick little salad of green ruffle-leaved lettuce, sliced cucumbers, and just-ripe 'Celebrity' tomatoes, dressed with a lemon, mustard, honey, garlic, and pepper vinaigrette; the whole meal was quick, light, and refreshing.

½ cup olive oil
¼ cup lemon juice
¼ cup chopped fresh basil, or
   1 tablespoon dried
2 medium eggplants, peeled and cut
   into ¼-inch-thick slices

2 large zucchini, cut into ¼-inch-thick
   slices
4 garlic cloves, thinly sliced
Salt and freshly milled black pepper

Pairing Vegetables and Herbs

Here are some common combinations; but don't let this list restrain you.

Basil: most famously with tomatoes, but also squash, peas, onions, potatoes
Chervil: beets, eggplant, peas, spinach, tomatoes
Chives: potatoes, especially with baked potatoes and sour cream
Dill: cucumbers, beets, turnips, potatoes, parsnips
Mint: peas, carrots, cabbage, fruit
Parsley: potatoes, carrots, tomatoes
Oregano and marjoram: carrots, peas, mushrooms, spinach, zucchini, dried beans, and in tomato
   sauces
Rosemary: potatoes, cauliflower, green beans, winter squash
Sage: carrots, eggplant, dried beans, winter squash
Thyme: asparagus, beans, beets, onions, zucchini

Combine the oil, lemon juice, and basil in a large bowl. Add the eggplant, zucchini, and garlic. Set aside for 15 minutes.

Preheat the broiler. Arrange the eggplant and zucchini slices on the broiler pan, leaving the garlic in the oil; sprinkle with salt and pepper. Broil for about 3 minutes, or until lightly browned. Turn the slices; drizzle with some of the oil from the bowl and top with the garlic slices; sprinkle with salt and pepper. Broil for about 3 minutes, or until tender and lightly browned.

TARRAGON CARROTS

MAKES 8 SERVINGS

At Ash Grove Community Farm in Corning, New York, Dori Green grows more than two hundred varieties of vegetables, herbs, fruits, and flowers (most open-pollinated, many heirlooms) on six chemical-free acres in an experimental raised-bed agroforestry structure. She also maintains ten acres managed for wildlife and medicinal herbs and berries, and four acres of pastures and orchards. Dori also raises free-range poultry and goats (the goats are also free-range too darned often, she says, but it seems a fence has to be watertight to hold them in if they see their feathered buddies on the other side).

4 cups small peeled carrots or large carrots cut into 3-inch pieces
¼ cup tarragon vinegar
2 tablespoons sugar
2 tablespoons chopped fresh parsley
2 tablespoons chopped green onion
1 teaspoon chopped fresh tarragon
½ teaspoon salt
Freshly milled black pepper

Cook the carrots in salted boiling water to cover in a medium saucepan until they are just tender, about 8 minutes; drain. Combine the vinegar, sugar, parsley, green onion, tarragon, ½ teaspoon salt, and pepper to taste and pour it over the drained, cooked carrots while they are still warm.

Cover the mixture and refrigerate it overnight. Drain the carrots well and pack them in a container with a tight-fitting lid.

BUTTERNUT-SAGE SQUASH

MAKES SIX SIDE-DISH SERVINGS

Hannah Bennett, a Kansas native, is an art major and a creative chef who cooks for and impresses her fellow farmworkers at Angelic Organics in Caledonia, Illinois, without ever looking at a recipe. Recently, Hannah served this roasted squash for a fall lunch along with a celeriac salad, Cheddar cheese, and good bread. She likes the versatility of roasted vegetables with herbs, and often alternates the vegetables and seasonings for variety.

1 (3-pound) butternut squash
2 tablespoons olive oil
1/4 cup chopped fresh sage

Kosher salt and freshly milled black pepper

Preheat the oven to 400°F. To prepare the squash, cut in half lengthwise. Remove and discard the seeds and strings. Peel the skin off the squash using a good vegetable peeler or a paring knife. Cut the squash into crescent-shaped slices about one-quarter inch thick.

Place the squash in a baking dish. Drizzle with the oil and sprinkle with the sage and salt and pepper.

Bake for about 45 minutes, or until the squash is tender but not mushy. Adjust the seasoning and serve.

NOTE: This recipe is delightfully simple, but it can be made only with very fresh butternut squash. If the squash is older and dried out, the flesh will not soften properly.

Meet the Farmers

Many Hands Organic Farm, Barre, Massachusetts

Julie Rawson grew up on a hog farm in Milledgeville, Illinois, about 130 miles west of Chicago. It was there that Julie's mother taught her about organic gardening and canning and preserving food. "I was seventeen by the time I started gardening on my own and she had already indoctrinated me," Julie recalls with a laugh. Her mother first got interested in organic gardening because of health concerns, but Julie says she also felt that "treating the earth appropriately" was an issue.

As a young adult, Julie left the farm to pursue a life in Chicago and then Boston, where she worked in the nonprofit world of community organizing. After Julie met Jack Kittredge, they decided they wanted to have a family in the country. The couple settled on fifty-five acres of land carved out of the rocky countryside of central Massachusetts, where they raised four children. These days, they intensely farm on about eight of the acres. The farm has been certified organic since 1987, only one year after the state began its organic certification program.

Through the years, they had heard about the CSA concept and were intrigued. Until it became a CSA in 1992, the farm sold its produce at a farmers' market, but the unpredictable demand made running the farm's business difficult. "In the old days, we'd have to guess what we could sell and it didn't always fit what people were looking for," Julie recalls. "It seemed like the whole town of Worcester would go on vacation in August and I couldn't sell anything just when I had the most crops."

Julie thinks CSAs have provided a wonderful link between people and their food. "When you're in a CSA, you have to learn how to use food—how to preserve it and use what you have instead of what you want," Julie says. "You can thank the CSA movement more than anything else for getting people interested in providing sustenance for themselves."

Julie's favorite crop is lettuce. The cool central Massachusetts nights and one-thousand-foot altitude make it possible to grow lettuce nearly straight through the summer so long as Julie starts new seedlings every week. Julie, who hates to waste things, particularly likes the fact that you can harvest the whole plant.

Herb Stuffings

Thanksgiving is a time of tradition, and for many families, sage stuffing is the only way to stuff a turkey. Here's a general recipe for it and a few herbal variations for those whose traditions are a bit more flexible:

Prepare about 8 cups of 1-inch bread cubes; use stale white bread, or if you don't have stale bread, leave the unwrapped bread on the counter for a few hours until it's stiff enough to cut into 1-inch cubes. In a large skillet, melt 1 tablespoon unsalted butter and sauté 1 medium onion (diced) and 1 cup chopped celery until the onion has wilted completely. Add the bread cubes, 3 cups of liquid (milk, stock, or a combination of the two), 2 teaspoons salt, 1 teaspoon freshly milled black pepper, and 2 to 3 tablespoons crumbled sage. If desired, add about 8 ounces of crumbled fried bacon or cooked sausage, and/or a chopped apple. Mix to thoroughly moisten the bread, then use the mixture to stuff a large turkey or bake it in a buttered casserole.

You can substitute another flavor for the sage—thyme, rosemary, or basil are just different enough to keep things interesting. Or, make a clean break and try a stuffing with a whole new taste:

Fennel, dried tomatoes, and cream with rye stuffing
Jalapeño pepper and cilantro with corn bread stuffing
Rosemary and shallots with wild rice stuffing
Pine nuts and oregano with Italian semolina bread stuffing
Lemon and thyme with brown rice stuffing

SOUR-CREAM CHIVE BREAD

MAKES 2 8-INCH LOAVES

This recipe was created in the kitchen of Boston's Food Project by some teenage interns in coordination with the project's chef/kitchen manager. These young people have all farmed in a core seven-week summer program as well as in an academic-year program. If they choose to stay with the project, they can apply to "apprentice" with a staff mentor in a specific area of work. During the summer program, the youths work on the farm to produce sustainably grown vegetables (and some fruits), which are distributed to their CSA and to an inner-city farmers' market. More than half the produce is donated to soup kitchens, food pantries, and shelters in the Boston area. Young people also serve in the shelters to which the Food Project donates its produce.

1 ½ cups all-purpose flour
1 ½ cups whole wheat flour
2 teaspoons baking powder
1 teaspoon baking soda
2 teaspoons salt
4 large eggs

2 cups sour cream
1 cup buttermilk
1 cup chives
½ cup sugar
3 tablespoons unsalted butter
2 teaspoons garlic

Preheat the oven to 350°F. Grease two 8-inch loaf pans.

Stir together the white and wheat flours, baking powder, baking soda, and salt. Beat the eggs in a separate bowl. Fold the sour cream, buttermilk, chives, sugar, butter, and garlic into the eggs.

Divide the batter into the greased loaf pans. Bake until brown and the centers spring back when gently pressed, about 40 minutes.

Tips on Using Fresh Herbs

- Snip fresh herbs with sharp scissors inside a paper bag to keep the small pieces from flying away.
- Heavy herbs, like rosemary and garlic, can withstand long cooking and can be added at the beginning of the cooking process. But more delicate herbs—basil, oregano, thyme, sage—deteriorate and can either lose flavor or become bitter when they're cooked for a long time. Add them only in the last 5 or 10 minutes of cooking (even if the recipe states otherwise).
- When using herbs in salad dressings, make the dressing an hour before using to allow the herbs to infuse the oil with flavor. Dress the salad just before serving, to keep the greens from becoming soggy.
- You can substitute fresh herbs for dried in almost any recipe; just use three or four times as much fresh as you would dried, because drying concentrates the flavor.
- The flavor of some herbs, particularly sage, thyme, and basil, intensifies when they are blanched or sautéed briefly.
- Herbs are potent; don't overseason by mixing too many of them or using too much. You can sometimes correct an overseasoned dish by straining out some of the herbs or adding more of less flavorful ingredients (like potatoes, rice, or squash).

Teas and Tonics

Humans have been steeping fragrant leaves and flowers in boiling water to produce tea for the past few millennia. Legend has it that Confucius invented tea so that his disciples would boil their water before drinking it.

To make a proper pot of tea, you need a pot made of china or pottery; a metal pot won't do (though you can boil the water in a metal kettle). Start with fresh, cold water and bring it to a rolling boil. Place about 2 tablespoons of fresh herbs or 1 tablespoon of dried herbs in your pot and pour the boiling water over them. Let the tea steep for about 5 minutes, then taste. Allow it to steep longer if you want it stronger. When it's strong enough, strain it with a tea strainer or through cheesecloth and pour it into cups; honey, lemon, chopped fresh herbs, candied flowers, and lemon peel are good accompaniments. Here are some herbs that make good tea:

- Basil, thyme, and fennel are good for digestive problems.
- Borage is a nice pick-me-up tea.
- Hyssop has a strong licorice flavor.
- Rosemary is used in the treatment of colds and headaches.
- Sage makes a full-bodied tea that can be used as a tonic and for fevers.

Mix sweet, citrusy, and distinctive flavors to create your own personal teas. For example, steep a lemony herb—lemon verbena, lemon balm, lemon basil—with fresh ginger and hyssop. Or add a few sprigs of rosemary to purchased exotic teas. Mint is a common tea ingredient and fresh mint makes it even better; try flavored mints (apple, orange, chocolate).

This recipe was created by Karen Shepherd, who owns and farms (with Tim Hermann) Blackberry Hills Farm in Wheeler, Wisconsin. She started with a recipe she loved as a child and made it healthier by substituting carob and raw honey for processed ingredients. She added peppermint because it had worked so well in a carob-rice dish.

CAROB-PEPPERMINT COOKIES

MAKES 48 COOKIES

⅔ cup raw carob powder, or ⅓ cup
   roasted
1 cup unsalted raw nut butter
½ cup honey
½ cup comb honey

⅓ cup safflower oil
2 cups rolled oats
½ cup dark raisins
¼ cup finely chopped fresh
   peppermint, or ⅛ cup dried

Mix the carob powder, nut butter, honeys, and oil over low heat and stir until bubbly. Stir in the oats, raisins, and peppermint and remove from the heat. Drop by the spoonful onto an oiled cookie sheet and put in the freezer. Serve frozen or slightly thawed.

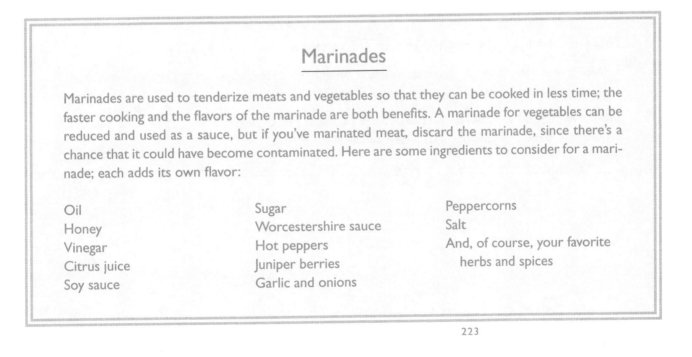

Marinades

Marinades are used to tenderize meats and vegetables so that they can be cooked in less time; the faster cooking and the flavors of the marinade are both benefits. A marinade for vegetables can be reduced and used as a sauce, but if you've marinated meat, discard the marinade, since there's a chance that it could have become contaminated. Here are some ingredients to consider for a marinade; each adds its own flavor:

Oil
Honey
Vinegar
Citrus juice
Soy sauce

Sugar
Worcestershire sauce
Hot peppers
Juniper berries
Garlic and onions

Peppercorns
Salt
And, of course, your favorite
   herbs and spices

Classic Combinations

Over the centuries, some herbs have been combined for specific uses or have become associated with regional cuisines. Among them:

Bouquet garni is a bundle of herbs—usually parsley, thyme, and bay leaf, but you can add others to your taste—that is tied together with string or enclosed in cheesecloth so that it is easy to remove from a soup or stew.

Fines herbes is used in egg and cheese dishes (it makes a very special omelet) and sauces. To make fines herbes, finely mince equal parts of chervil, parsley, tarragon, and thyme and add at the very last minute.

Herbes de Provence is a blend of thyme, rosemary, sage, basil, and marjoram that adds a hint of the south of France to sauces, stews, and sautéed vegetables. It's a good addition to marinades and salad dressings.

Herbes Italianos, a blend of oregano, thyme, bay leaves, basil, sage, and peppercorns, imparts the flavor of Italy. It is wonderful on pizzas and in ratatouilles.

Zatar is a Middle Eastern mix of thyme, sumac, parsley, sesame seeds, and olive oil.

Adobe seasoning is great in guacamole and on grilled vegetables and chicken. It's made from garlic, onion, Mexican oregano, cumin, and hot peppers.

Thai, the classic herb-and-spice blend, is bell peppers, garlic, ginger, black pepper, hot peppers, lemongrass, basil, and cilantro, plus a rare spice called galangal.

CHAPTER ELEVEN

COOKING WITH FRUIT

There is no comparison between the farm-fresh fruit distributed at CSA sites and the travel-weary possibilities available in neighborhood markets. Often the colorful shares of apples, berries, melons, nectarines, peaches, and pears attract passersby on the sidewalk, and they stay to learn more about the CSA and become members. There is really not very much that you need to know when your fruit comes from a CSA. Just hours from the plant, bush, or tree, the fruit is ripe, flavorful, and ready to use. It is often so enticing that it's all eaten by the time you get home. If not, the recipes that follow are some of our favorite ways to use what's left.

Ripening

All fruits undergo changes after harvest that affect the length of time they can be stored. Some fruits can ripen after they have been picked and others can't. While ripening on the plant, bush, or tree is desirable for full flavor development, apples, apricots, avocados, bananas, peaches, pears, plums, and many tropical fruits can ripen once picked, particularly in the presence of ethylene gas, which is released by other ripening fruits in the process. Cherries, citrus fruits, figs, grapes, melons, pineapple, and strawberries cannot ripen after they are harvested. The changes that they undergo are related to deterioration.

The first thing to do when you arrive home with your share or purchase of fresh fruit is to determine its ripeness. Most fruit is best if stored at cool room temperature rather than in the refrigerator, until it has reached its peak of ripeness. Then it should be prepared and served or refrigerated to prolong the period before it becomes overripe. Fruits, especially fragile ones such as berries, cherries, and apricots, will keep longer if not rinsed until you are ready to use them. Any moisture on the surface of the fruit will cause it to soften quickly. An open bowl, a brown paper bag, or a "breathable" plastic bag that is made especially for produce is the best choice for storing fruits that can ripen after they are picked (see Ripening, page 225) rather than a tight container that will trap the ethylene gas they produce and cause them to overripen quickly.

Preparing Fruit

Prepare fruit to be served raw as close to serving time as possible so that sliced fruit doesn't dry out or become brown from oxidation, and so that berries and cherries don't soften from rinsing. If it is necessary to slice apples, apricots, bananas, peaches, pears, plums, or nectarines more than a few minutes before serving, toss them in a little citrus juice to retard browning from oxidation. When slicing fruit, be sure to use a stainless steel knife so that the metal doesn't react with the acid in the fruit and discolor it.

Cooking fruit can avoid some of these problems. Cooking retards browning and intentionally causes softening so that fruits that are cooked before serving can be prepared several hours ahead and stored, covered, in the refrigerator. It is still best to rinse, peel, or slice them just before cooking so that changes don't occur before they are cooked. Cooking has often been used as a method of preservation for fruit. Canning cooked fruits, fruit purees, jams, jellies, preserves, and pickles makes it possible to save an abundant crop at its peak and to enjoy the summertime flavor of fruit all year long.

Judie Caporiccio, who farms Wild Iris Farm in West Richland, Washington, admits that she couldn't run her farm without her members' help. Member Toby Swanger submitted this recipe for strawberry bread. She likes to make it with whole wheat flour for both the flavor and the fiber it provides.

²⁄₃ cup chopped pecans (optional)
1²⁄₃ cups unbleached all-purpose or
  whole wheat flour (see Note)
¾ cup sugar
1 teaspoon ground cinnamon
½ teaspoon baking soda

½ teaspoon salt
2 large eggs
½ cup vegetable oil
1 cup small fresh strawberries, thinly
  sliced

Preheat the oven to 350°F. Grease an 8-inch loaf pan. If using the pecans, spread them out on a rimmed cookie sheet and toast for 3 to 5 minutes in the 350°F oven.

Combine the flour, sugar, pecans, if using, cinnamon, baking soda, and salt in a large bowl.

Whisk the eggs in a small bowl until frothy; whisk in the oil. Make a well in the center of the flour mixture and pour in the egg mixture. Blend just until the dry ingredients are moistened. Fold in the strawberries.

Spoon the mixture into the prepared pan and smooth the top. Bake for 45 to 60 minutes, until a cake tester inserted in the center comes out clean. Let cool in the pan for 5 minutes; remove and let cool on a wire rack.

NOTE: Or, use a combination of the two.

SUMMER STRAWBERRY BREAD

MAKES 1 8-INCH LOAF

WATERMELON, ARUGULA, RED ONION, AND VELLA DRY SALAD

MAKES 8 SERVINGS

This recipe was contributed by John McReynolds of the Café La Haye in Sonoma, California. The artisanal dry Jack cheese called for in this recipe is available in gourmet stores nationally and is worth a search. If you can't find it, you can substitute Parmigiano-Reggiano.

2 red onions, very thinly sliced
1/4 teaspoon salt
Citrus Vinaigrette (recipe follows)
2 pounds watermelon, cut into small cubes (about 2 cups)

1 pound arugula, rinsed, drained, and trimmed
Freshly milled black pepper
8 ounces Vella dry Jack cheese, shaved

Combine the onions and salt in a colander placed in a bowl and set aside for 30 minutes. Rinse the onions and place in ice water until ready to serve. Meanwhile, prepare the citrus vinaigrette.

To serve, combine the watermelon, arugula, onions, and salt and pepper to taste in a large bowl; toss with 1/2 cup citrus vinaigrette. Mound the salad on chilled plates. Top with the cheese.

CITRUS VINAIGRETTE: Combine 4 shallots, finely chopped, 1/4 cup orange juice, 1/4 cup Champagne vinegar, 2 tablespoons lemon juice, 3 tablespoons grated orange peel or 1 tablespoon grated lemon peel, and salt and pepper to taste in a small bowl. Gradually whisk in 1/2 cup canola oil and 1/4 cup extra-virgin olive oil. Whisk again before using. Makes 2 cups.

CITRUS COLLARDS WITH RAISINS

MAKES 2 SERVINGS

Here's a sweet, modern twist to this traditional southern "soul food" favorite. Bryant Terry of the Park Slope CSA in Brooklyn, New York (which gets vegetables from Cooke Hollow Farm in Valley Falls), submitted this recipe.

1 large bunch collard greens
Coarse sea salt
1/2 tablespoon extra-virgin olive oil

1 garlic clove, minced
1/3 cup raisins
2 medium oranges

Remove the stems from the collards and discard. Stack four or five leaves on top of one another. Roll the leaves into a tight cylinder. Slice crosswise, cutting the leaves into thin strips. Rinse the leaves in cold water and drain in a colander.

In a large pot over high heat, bring 3 quarts water to a boil and add 3 teaspoons salt. Add the collards and cook, uncovered, for 10 minutes. Remove, drain, and plunge into a bowl of ice water to stop the cooking and set the color of the greens. Drain.

In a medium sauté pan, over medium heat, warm the oil. Add the garlic and sauté for 1 minute. Add the collards, raisins, and a pinch of salt. Sauté for 3 minutes, stirring frequently. Section the oranges, reserving the juice. Add the oranges and juice and cook for an additional 30 seconds. Do not overcook (collards should be bright green).

Serve immediately or at room temperature.

GOLDEN HONEYDEW *PICO DE GALLO*

MAKES 6 SERVINGS

Chef Ben Schulman of Exxon Mobil Headquarters on Bell Street in Houston told us that he updated the flavor of *pico de gallo* by incorporating some locally grown and newly harvested golden honeydew from the Houston farmers' market with some of the other, more "traditional" ingredients to make a topping for the Chipotle-Chile Barbecued Snapper that he entered in the Culinary Challenge 2001 in that city. We found it to be a delicious accompaniment to any seafood, and to poultry.

6 large ripe plum tomatoes, chopped
6 large tomatillos, chopped
4 jalapeño peppers, chopped
2 large red onions, chopped

1 cup 1/4-inch cubes golden honeydew
    melon
1 bunch fresh cilantro, chopped
1/3 cup lime juice
Salt

Combine the tomatoes, tomatillos, jalapeño peppers, onions, and honeydew in a large bowl. Fold in the cilantro, lime juice, and salt to taste. Cover and refrigerate for at least 2 hours before serving.

- All fruit, especially berries, will keep longer if not washed until ready to serve.
- To speed up ripening in those fruits that will ripen after harvest, put the fruit in a tight container with an apple or a pear.
- Many fruits will discolor when peeled or cut due to exposure to oxygen. To inhibit this, dip them in lemon or other citrus juice, keep them submerged in water or a syrup, or brush them with one of the commercial antioxidant products.

QUICK CURRANT BREAD PUDDING

MAKES 4 SERVINGS

In Great Britain, this pretty dessert is known as Summer Pudding. We developed this easy version, served at room temperature, to use the red currants we got in our July fruit shares.

1 cup red currants
⅔ cup orange juice
⅓ cup sugar
2 tablespoons lemon juice
16 thin slices firm white bread, crusts removed

½ cup red or black raspberries, blueberries, or sliced fresh strawberries
Whipped cream (sweetened or not) or crème fraîche

Bring the currants, orange juice, and sugar to a full boil over medium heat, stirring until the sugar is dissolved. Remove from the heat and stir in the lemon juice.

Cut 8 slices of the bread diagonally in half and cut a 2¾-inch round from each of 4 slices. Chop the trimmings and the remaining 4 bread slices.

Spoon 1 tablespoon currant mixture into each of four 6-ounce (¾ cup) custard cups or individual soufflé dishes. Reserve ⅓ cup currant mixture for garnish. Combine the chopped bread with the remaining currant mixture and the raspberries.

Swirl the custard cups to moisten the sides of each cup with currant syrup. Fit 4 bread triangles into each custard cup with the 90-degree angles meeting in the center and the tops overlapping as necessary. Divide the raspberry mixture among the cups. Trim off any points of bread extending more than

Meet the Farmers

Molly's Island Garden, Langley, Washington

In 1987, Molly and John Petersons moved to their farm on Whidbey Island, the largest island in Puget Sound, located across from Seattle. They started growing and selling their produce at the farmers' market within a year. As they were always looking for new and stable markets for their bounty, they decided to start their CSA in 1993. "It just makes a lot of sense," Molly says. "To have produce wasted because of factors you have no control over is disappointing." Anna, the Petersons' daughter, grew up on the farm. She has returned to run the farm and manage the CSA. While Molly also works for domestic violence victim services and John works for the state, Anna, twenty, runs the CSA and the farm full-time and hopes she always will. "I hope to be doing it the rest of my life," Anna says.

Anna believes corporate agriculture exploits not only the land but the people who work it. Molly's Island Garden now has one part-time employee. The woman works in the fields with her baby nestled on her back for five to ten hours a week, as her schedule permits. Though the Petersons have no plans to increase the number of shareholders, Anna believes such a move could benefit the community economically. "As much as I hate the idea of just managing other people, I do think this community could use more farmers rather than Dairy Queen employees," she says.

The Petersons have an adventurous group of shareholders who are always up for trying new varieties of vegetables. The family aims to meet the demand—indeed, this season they're growing ten to fifteen different kinds of tomatoes after swearing off the crop for several years in the wake of a tomato blight. They've also found that a splash of unexpected color on traditional vegetables also wakes up the appetite. So, their fields are teeming with at least fifteen types of purple vegetables ranging from purple string beans to purple potatoes to purple cauliflower. "People just want something that the Joneses don't have, but they don't want it to taste too strange," Anna says.

⅛ inch above the filling and add the scraps to the filling. Top each pudding with a bread round. Press down on the puddings with the bottom of a drinking glass to compress and flatten the surface.

To serve, loosen the edges of each pudding with a kitchen knife and unmold onto a serving plate; drizzle each with some of the remaining ⅓ cup currant mixture and serve with whipped cream.

BLUEBERRY CAKE

MAKES 9 SERVINGS

Susan Butterworth of Marblehead, Massachusetts, a member of the Marblehead Eco-Farm/Direct Co-op, gave us this recipe for her mother's Blueberry Cake along with this memory: "Our family spent two weeks every summer at Lake Wentworth in Wolfeboro, New Hampshire, in the late 1950s and early 1960s. We would pile into the station wagon, the old 1954 Ford, loaded with boxes of bedding, swimming gear, board games, and children's books. Days would be spent swimming in the lake, but often in the evening we'd pack a picnic and drive to a hiking spot for supper. One was a small mountain called Tumbledown Dick, which had a wonderful blueberry patch. We'd pick and eat, and the next day Mom would make Blueberry Cake."

1 cup all-purpose flour
1 teaspoon baking powder
1/4 teaspoon salt
2 large eggs, separated
1 cup vegetable shortening

1 cup sugar
1/3 cup milk
1 teaspoon vanilla extract
1 cup blueberries

Preheat the oven to 375°F. Grease and flour a 9-inch square baking pan. Sift together the flour, baking powder, and salt.

Beat the egg whites with an electric mixer and set them aside. With the same beaters, beat the shortening with the sugar; beat in the egg yolks. Alternately add the milk and dry ingredients to the shortening mixture. Fold in the egg whites and vanilla. Add the blueberries and pour the mixture into the pan.

Bake for 25 to 30 minutes, until a toothpick inserted in the center comes out dry (except for the blueberry juice!).

Reuben Haag is the executive chef for Bon Appétit in Clinton, New York, where he oversees the food served at all of Hamilton College's cafeterias and catered events. Reuben seeks out local produce when possible because locally grown bell peppers, apples, corn, and tomatoes not only taste fresher but are also generally less expensive in season. "In the fall I can get five different varieties of local apples and they're good-quality and less expensive than the polished ones from Washington State," he says. Reuben usually makes his blackberry cobbler in the summer when berries are more plentiful. Reuben recommends that the cobbler, once baked, be allowed to set for about 15 minutes before cutting. This prevents the juices from running too much.

BLACKBERRY COBBLER

MAKES 6 SERVINGS

4 to 5 cups blackberries
1/2 cup plus 2 tablespoons sugar
1 1/2 tablespoons quick-cooking tapioca
9 tablespoons unsalted butter
1 cup all-purpose flour

1 1/2 teaspoons baking powder
1/4 teaspoon salt
1/4 cup milk
1 large egg, lightly beaten
Vanilla ice cream (optional)

Toss together the blackberries, the 1/2 cup sugar, the tapioca, and 1 tablespoon of the butter in a medium saucepan and set aside for about 10 minutes to moisten the tapioca. Lightly grease a 1 1/2-quart casserole.

Meanwhile, stir together the flour, the 2 tablespoons sugar, the baking powder, and the salt. Cut in the remaining 8 tablespoons butter with a pastry blender or two knives. In a separate bowl, combine the milk and egg. Add all at once to the dry ingredients and stir only until combined. Be careful not to overmix.

Preheat the oven to 400°F. Cook the blackberry mixture over low heat, stirring until it comes to a full boil, about 10 minutes.

Pour the blackberry mixture into the casserole and spoon the topping over all. Bake for 20 to 25 minutes, until the cobbler is golden brown. Serve warm with vanilla ice cream, if desired.

FINNISH BERRY RICE

MAKES 4 TO 6 SERVINGS

Grindstone Farm in Pulaski, New York, prides itself on "excellence in edible, incredible organics" (which they usually refer to as "E.I.E.I.O"). They've developed their own definition and standard of organic growing as a system that "allows only natural enrichment of the soil life, avoiding all synthetic chemicals and pesticides." They employ companion planting, crop rotation, improvement of the soils with manures, composts, mulches, and cover crops. Grindstone Farm also uses Integrated Pest Management (IPM), rotates crops between fields to keep pests from building up and to improve soil life, and selects bushes and flowers to attract beneficial insects for their predatory abilities against unwanted pests. Grindstone's organic farming produces nutrient-rich, healthy soil to feed its plants and maintain healthy water quality.

1 cup heavy cream
1/4 cup sugar
2 cups raspberries, blueberries,
   or halved strawberries

2 to 3 cups cooked rice, chilled
Fresh mint leaves

Beat the cream until soft peaks form. Gradually add the sugar and beat until stiff.

Fold the cream and 1 cup of the berries into the rice. Spoon into a serving dish and top with the remaining 1 cup berries and the mint leaves.

Marilyn Isom's Autumn Lane Farm is the first CSA farm in the Springfield, Missouri, area. To introduce the concept to the community, she has offered incentives, advertised, and is working with other organic growers to form a growers' co-op that matches farms with chefs and restaurants. The jams Marilyn has developed to use the fruit from her cherry and pear trees are family favorites. This pear jam was created to use a bumper crop of pears one year; the Isoms love the unusual tastes of the ginger and (see Variation) the five-spice powder. Pear jam is a good accompaniment to beef and poultry dishes.

GINGERED PEAR JAM

MAKES ABOUT 6 HALF-PINTS

5 1/2 cups sugar

4 cups chopped pears, peeled, cored, and finely chopped

2 tablespoons lemon juice

1/2 teaspoon unsalted butter or margarine

2 teaspoons grated peeled fresh ginger

1 box powdered pectin

Sterilize jars, lids, and rings; bring about 6 inches water to a boil in a water-bath canner. Measure sugar into a medium bowl. Place pears in the bowl of a food processor fitted with a chopping blade and pulse to chop. Combine chopped pears, lemon juice, butter, and ginger in an 8-quart sauce pot. Stir in pectin and bring to a full rolling boil over high heat. Add sugar and boil 1 minute, stirring constantly. Remove sauce pot from heat; skim off any foam and ladle into sterilized jars filling to within 1/8 inch of the top. Add lids and rings and process in a boiling water bath, 10 minutes.

VARIATION: Substitute 1 tablespoon Asian five-spice powder for the ginger.

CHAPTER TWELVE

BEYOND PRODUCE

For many people, the words "organic" and "agriculture" conjure up images of leafy greens, ripe tomatoes, and juicy apples. Indeed, over 50 percent of the organic products raised in the United States are fruits and vegetables. But more and more farmers and consumers are realizing that many other farm-raised products contribute to the condition of our environment—and that if these products are raised thoughtfully and sustainably, they not only are healthier in both the long and short runs, but also taste better. That's why many CSA farms, to the delight of their members, offer a wide range of foods (and some nonedibles) that don't grow in the ground.

Poultry and Eggs

Most people who know anything about the commercial poultry industry know that we don't want to think too much about how chickens are raised. Conditions are atrocious both for the chickens and for us and result in poultry and eggs that are often contaminated with bacteria. To combat this, large poultry farms regularly add antibiotics to their chicken feed, which is passed on to us when we eat these chickens. The medical profession has warned us that the antibiotics we consume in our poultry is creating resistant strains of bacteria.

That's why Jay and Polly Armour of Four Winds Farm in Gardiner, New York, raise their chickens and turkeys in movable shelters on open pasture. They say, "By moving these shelters daily, the birds have access to fresh air, sunshine, and, most important, a clean, fresh 'salad bar' regularly. These healthy, vigorous birds don't need the constant doses of medication that are required in conventional poultry-confinement operations. The result is cleaner and healthier chickens and eggs, as well as tastier ones." Eggs offered at CSAs come in a pretty palette of colors—white, brown, cream, and even pale blue—because the farms raise a diverse group of chickens (different breeds lay different color eggs). Many members relate that every dish cooked with these eggs tastes better.

Meat and Dairy

Every problem associated with poultry and eggs affects meat and dairy products as well. Bovine growth hormones, which are passed into milk, have had little testing—no one really knows how they'll affect us after we've consumed them for thirty or forty years. And the factory farms where most livestock is raised are cruel environments where animals are kept in pens and fed a diet of grain that produces meat with a high percentage of saturated fat.

Grass-fed beef, such as that raised at Peaceful Pastures in Hickman, Tennessee, and Tir na nOg Farm in Walton, New York, is leaner and higher in omega-3 fatty acids ("good" fat that is required for cell development). Chefs and home cooks alike are discovering another advantage to responsibly raised livestock: Grass-fed beef is more tender and cooks faster and more evenly.

Dairy products such as fresh goat cheese and artisanal cheeses are hard to find, but many CSAs offer them.

Seafood

Americans have tripled their consumption of fish in the past thirty years, spurred by health and environmental concerns. Unfortunately, this has led to a whole new set of problems. Fish farming has produced abundant and cheap supplies—but the process is fouling waters all over the world. And our oceans are being overfished to the point where certain species are endangered.

The situation is confusing: For some fish, such as salmon, we're advised to use only wild-caught fish. For others, we're told to look for farm-raised. There are even distinctions for different methods of fishing. Some CSAs offer fish from responsible sources. Several organizations, including Chefs Collaborative, are distributing lists that divide seafood into recommended, not-so-recommended, and try-to-avoid categories (see pages 242–43).

Honey and Maple Syrup

The Northeast has been plagued by a shortage of pollinating bees, so farmers often install hives near their crops, which leads to a delightful bonus for CSA members: fresh honey with a taste that varies depending on which flowers the bees browsed. Clover honey is especially tasty, but it's always nice to note the differences in each batch. Maple syrup is another "CSA extra," an agricultural product that many farms use to supplement income.

And More

Farmers and members often suggest other products that the farmers or other local small businesses can provide. CSAs that raise sheep offer wool yarn or beautifully woven blankets. Some farms raise and mill quinoa, an ancient South American grain that contains complete protein. Natural soaps and lotions that contain olive oil, goat milk, or flowers—they lather luxuriantly—are always a hit.

EGGS IN TOMATO NESTS

MAKES 1 SERVING

At Boann's Banks, in Royston, Georgia, Chris and Eric Wagoner raise heirloom and open-pollinated vegetables and free-range hens. They note major differences between their eggs and the ones found in supermarkets: "The most obvious difference (besides the wonderful taste) is the color of the yolk. A hen with access to green grass and plenty of bugs produces eggs with yolks that are vividly yellow, nearly orange. Hens that spend their lives in cages produce a pale yolk whose color is largely derived from marigold petals and other coloring agents mixed in the feed. The rich color from our eggs will do wonders for your recipes, too—cake batter, homemade ice cream, omelets, and deviled eggs will all be the color they were meant to be. You'll notice a difference in the freshness, too. Our eggs will have been laid no more than a week before you buy them. Fresh eggs have a much firmer white, resulting in thicker fried and poached eggs. The yolk is also firmer and more resistant to breaking, making sunny-side-up eggs a breeze to cook. Many restaurants specifically request older eggs because their fried eggs look larger on the plate or sandwich, since they run out into the skillet. One instance where you really do want them older is for hard-cooked eggs. You've probably noticed when peeling eggs that under the shell are two distinct skins (the air pocket is between these two layers). In fresh eggs, the bond between these two is very tight, and that makes peeling very difficult. If you plan on making a large number of hard-cooked eggs for Easter or deviled eggs or whatever, buy them a couple weeks in advance and let them age in your refrigerator. Peeling will be much easier."

To answer another frequently asked question: Why are some of the Wagoners' eggs green? They're from Araucana hens, a breed descended from a flock kept by a Peruvian tribe found a century ago. Inside, they're the same as the others.

You can multiply this recipe by the number of people you are serving and use the larger amounts if you want to serve two eggs per person. The baking instructions are the same no matter how many you do.

1 or 2 medium heirloom tomatoes
1 or 2 teaspoons unsalted butter
1 or 2 eggs

Salt and freshly milled black pepper
Shredded cheese (optional)
Chopped fresh parsley (optional)

Preheat the oven to 350°F. Lightly oil a baking dish large enough to hold the number of tomato nests you are preparing. Cut the top from each tomato and hollow out some of the center. Place 1 teaspoon butter in the cavity of each tomato. Crack 1 egg into the cavity. Sprinkle with salt and pepper. Place in the baking dish; top with shredded cheese and parsley, if using, and bake for 15 to 20 minutes, until the eggs are firm.

VANILLA CREAM PIE

MAKES 4 SERVINGS

Jenny Drake of Hickman, Tennessee's Peaceful Pastures begs forgiveness for this recipe from those who are careful about fat consumption. But this recipe brings out the best in the fresh milk, butter, cream, and eggs she raises, so she likes to indulge every once in a while!

¹/₂ cup plus 2 tablespoons sugar
¹/₄ cup cornstarch
¹/₈ teaspoon salt
5 large egg yolks, lightly beaten
2 cups whole milk
¹/₂ cup heavy cream

2 tablespoons unsalted butter
2 teaspoons vanilla extract
1 (9-inch) prebaked piecrust or graham cracker crust
Whipped cream

Whisk together the sugar, cornstarch, and salt in a medium saucepan. Add the yolks, then quickly whisk in the milk, cream, and butter. Cook, stirring constantly, over medium heat until thickened, 8 to 12 minutes. Remove the pan from the heat and stir in the vanilla.

Pour into the piecrust and chill. Top with whipped cream before serving.

VARIATION: For banana pudding, layer sliced ripe bananas and vanilla wafers in a large bowl and pour the filling over them. Top with whipped cream, if desired.

HAZELNUT COOLER

MAKES 1 SERVING

"Here is an absurdly simple recipe that is quick and astoundingly tasty, and, since we don't produce that many hazelnuts, a very good way to stretch their use," says Will Newman II of CSA at Natural Harvest Farm in the North Willamette Valley, near Portland, Oregon. A research project of Oregon Sustainable Agriculture Land Trust (OSALT), the CSA at Natural Harvest first began in 1988 with four shareholders. It grew until 1997, when the farm owners donated the farm to OSALT, a charitable nonprofit research and education organization dedicated to rediscovering and developing sustainable*

*OSALT, along with a number of other organizations, defines "sustainable" as "ecologically sound, economically practical, and socially equitable."

practices for the production and distribution of agricultural bounty (food, fiber, plants, and building materials). Natural Harvest is being developed as a demonstration and research site for the trust. The CSA operation is an education project as well: Each year the Natural Harvest site manager works with a young grower or two while they operate the CSA. OSALT provides technical assistance, access to the land and water, training, and advice. The researchers establish objectives for the year, operate the CSA, and produce a report at the end of the year summarizing their work, presenting the data and conclusions, and offering suggestions for further research by future CSA operators. (Other education activities are also conducted on the twenty-acre farm.) "We grow annual vegetables as well as a variety of tree fruits (apple, pear, plum, cherry, hazelnut/filbert, fig, Asian pear, quince, crab apple), perennial herbs, berries (blackberry, raspberry, boysenberry, Marionberry, gooseberry, blueberry, currant), and grapes (about twenty-five varieties for snacking and juice). Natural Harvest is home to about fifty ducks, honey and orchard mason bees, one sheep, and a llama. We are all allowed to live and do our work here by the six cats whose home this is," says Will.

6 to 8 roasted hazelnuts   *1 cup cow's milk, rice milk, or soy milk*

Put the nuts in a blender; chop them very small. Add the milk and mix well. Drink within a few minutes or remix.

Sea Watch

Environmental organizations on both coasts have contributed to the following lists of seafood to look for and those to avoid.

Best Choices

Abalone (farmed)
Catfish (U.S. farmed)
Caviar (farmed)
Clams (farmed)
Crab, Dungeness
Halibut (Pacific)
Hoki
Lobster, Rock (Calif., Australia)
Mussels (farmed)
Oysters (farmed)
Sablefish/Black Cod (Alaska, British Columbia)
Salmon (Calif., Alaska, wild-caught)

Salmon, canned
Sand Dabs
Sardines
Shrimp/Prawns (trap-caught)
Squid/Calamari (Calif. market squid)
Striped Bass (farmed)
Sturgeon (farmed)
Tilapia (farmed)
Tuna, Albacore
Tuna, canned white (Albacore)
Tuna, Yellowfin/Ahi (troll/pole-caught)

Proceed with Caution

Clams (wild-caught)
Cod, Pacific
Crab, Imitation, Surimi
Crab, King
Crab, Snow
Lobster, American
Mahimahi
Mussels (wild-caught)
Oysters (wild-caught)
Pollock
Sablefish/Black Cod (Calif., Wash., Oreg.)

Salmon (Oreg., Wash., wild-caught)
Scallops, Bay
Shark, Thresher (U.S. West Coast)
Shrimp (U.S., wild-caught)
Shrimp, Bay
Sole, English/Petrale/Dover
Swordfish (U.S. West Coast)
Trout, Rainbow (farmed)
Tuna, Yellowfin/Ahi
Tuna, canned chunk light

Avoid

Caviar, Beluga/Osetra/Sevruga	Salmon (farmed, Atlantic)
Chilean Sea Bass	Scallops, Sea
Cod, Atlantic/Icelandic	Sharks (except U.S. West Coast Thresher)
Lingcod	Shrimp (wild-caught or farmed)
Monkfish	Sturgeon (wild-caught)
Orange Roughy	Swordfish (Atlantic)
Rockfish/Rock Cod/Pacific Snapper	Tuna (Bluefin)

Meet the Farmers

Local Harvest, Wellman and Solon, Iowa

Simone Alvarez and Susan Zacharakis-Jutz became fast friends soon after they met and began discussing the idea of running a CSA together. Although they come from very different backgrounds and their farms are located a forty-five-minute drive from each other, their partnership has blossomed along with Local Harvest, the CSA they formed in 1997.

Simone, a native of France, was teaching French at the University of Iowa when she decided to retire early to manage her twenty-acre farm full-time. Susan had grown up milking cows on a conventional dairy farm in Minnesota, but it wasn't until 1993 that she and her husband, a community-development specialist with the Iowa State University Extension, decided to buy the eighty-acre farm they now live on with their children. In 1997, the two women put together a business plan. Their concept: Offer vegetable shares from Susan's farm and fresh bread, eggs, and flower shares from Simone's farm. The two have built a multiproducer CSA that is stronger than the sum of its parts. "Part of our goal from the start was to help individual producers have an outlet for their products. It's appealing for our members because it's sort of a one-stop shopping idea," Susan says. The CSA had about ninety-three vegetable share members in its 2002 season.

GRILLED RIB EYE STEAK WITH TAPENADE, ROASTED NEW POTATOES, AND BABY LEEKS

MAKES 4 SERVINGS

Michael Leviton is the chef and co-owner (with his wife, Jill) of Lumière, a restaurant in Newton, Massachusetts. Michael values his ongoing relationships with local farms including Dancing Bear Farm in nearby Leyden. The farm's high-quality fresh vegetables make it possible for Michael to prepare his favorite style of food: relatively simple. "They're delicious without the chef having to do more to derive flavor," Michael says. This recipe will be even tastier when prepared with natural hormone-free meats such as that offered by the Niman Ranch of Oakland, California. You can purchase the Niman Ranch meat online at www.nimanranch.com, or seek out local meat producers near your home.

2 tablespoons finely chopped anchovies
2 tablespoons finely chopped garlic
Olive oil
1 1/2 cups pitted oil-cured ripe olives
2 tablespoons finely chopped capers
2 tablespoons red wine vinegar
Freshly milled black pepper
16 baby red, white, or Yukon gold potatoes (about 1 1/2 inches in diameter), scrubbed
Salt
16 baby leeks
4 (8- to 10-ounce) rib eye steaks

Prepare the tapenade: Combine the anchovies and garlic in a small nonreactive saucepan. Barely cover with olive oil and cook over very low heat until the anchovies and garlic have essentially "melted" together and are incredibly soft. This will take about 30 to 45 minutes. Remove from the heat and let cool.

Combine the anchovy-garlic mixture with the olives, capers, and vinegar in a food processor or blender. Process until the mixture is homogenous but not completely smooth. Slowly add 1/4 to 1/2 cup olive oil, to taste. Adjust the seasoning with pepper to give it a little bit of a bite. Leave the tapenade a little loose (that is, with a bit more olive oil) so it can mix with the steak juices and become like a vinaigrette for the vegetables. Set aside.

Preheat the oven to 500°F. Cut the potatoes into 1/4- to 1/3-inch rounds; toss with 1 tablespoon olive oil and season with salt and pepper. Arrange the potatoes in a single layer on a sheet pan lined with parchment paper. Roast for 12 to 15 minutes, until lightly browned and tender. Set aside.

Trim the leeks to about 4 inches in length. Trim a thin slice from the root ends and split the leeks lengthwise almost to the bottom, leaving enough of the bases intact to hold them together. Rinse the leeks thoroughly in cool water and drain well. Toss the leeks with 1 tablespoon olive oil and season with salt and pepper. Lay the leeks in a single layer on a sheet pan lined with parchment paper. Roast the leeks for 10 minutes, or until lightly browned and tender at the bases. Set aside.

Season the steaks liberally with salt and pepper. Grill the steaks over high heat to the desired doneness, 3 to 5 minutes per side. Let the steaks rest for about 5 minutes, collecting any juices that are released. Mix the juices with the tapenade.

While the steaks are grilling, return the leeks and potatoes to the oven to warm them. When hot, divide the vegetables equally among 4 plates. Place the steaks on the plates and serve with the tapenade on the side.

RIVER RUN FARM MARINATED GARLIC CHUCK ROAST

MAKES 6 SERVINGS

River Run Farm in Clatskanie, Oregon, provides organic beef to local customers in the Northwest as well as by mail across the country.

I head garlic (about 15 cloves)
I (3- to 3½-pound) boneless grass-fed
    beef chuck roast
I large onion, finely chopped
½ cup strong freshly brewed coffee
¼ cup soy sauce

¼ cup Asian marinade and dipping
    sauce (see Note)
I tablespoon dry sherry
I tablespoon Worcestershire sauce
I tablespoon red wine vinegar
½ teaspoon ground ginger

Peel the garlic and sliver part of it. Cut slits in the meat with a small, sharp knife. Insert the slivered garlic deep into the slits all over the roast. Finely chop the remaining garlic and mix with the onion, coffee, soy sauce, Asian marinade, sherry, Worcestershire sauce, vinegar, and ginger; pour over the roast. Cover and marinate in the refrigerator for at least 12 hours, turning several times.

Preheat an outdoor grill or the broiler. Remove the meat from the marinade. Bring the marinade to a boil in a small saucepan. Grill or broil the meat to the desired doneness (145°F for medium-rare, 160°F for medium), brushing frequently with the marinade. Slice thinly and serve.

NOTE: The chef recommends Yoshida's Original Gourmet Sauce.

Double Check Ranch occupies some ten thousand acres in Winkelman, Arizona, sixty miles north of Tucson. The ranch is dedicated to improving the watershed by practicing holistic management. Farmer Jean Schennesen provides her customers with natural, grass-fed beef, processed at a small packing house right on the ranch, and offers "Working Weekend on a Working Ranch" getaways.

1 to 1½ pounds beef strips or thinly
  sliced sirloin
1 medium onion, chopped
1 tablespoon vegetable oil
2 tablespoons soy sauce

½ cup sliced mushrooms
1 to 1½ cups ranch dressing
4 cups hot cooked rotini or other curly
  noodles

Brown the meat and onion slowly and gently in the oil, 6 to 8 minutes. Add the soy sauce and cook until somewhat absorbed, about 4 minutes. Add the mushrooms and cook until the meat, onion, and mushrooms are tender, 15 to 20 minutes. Add the dressing; heat until warmed through and serve over the hot noodles.

DOUBLE CHECK BEEF STROGANOFF

MAKES 4 SERVINGS

SCOTCH BROTH

Zach, Holly, and Bethany Shaltz, a "retired" military family, moved to Michigan in 1997 to build Shaltz Farm in Boyne City, which includes a small market garden, pigs for meat, chickens for eggs, and a flock of quality registered Shetland sheep. Each spring, a few Shetland lambs don't make the grade as breeding stock and are processed for meat. Shetland lambs have an extremely mild flavor and are smaller—so you don't have to invite all the relatives to sit down to a delicious leg-of-lamb dinner. The Schaltzes' Shetlands are pasture-raised, so their flavor is even better, and the meat leaner because they're not fed concentrates to create artificial weight gain. The Schaltzes vaccinate their sheep but don't use any other medications, hormones, or antibiotics. They also don't use any chemicals on their pasture, just green grass, blue sky, and yellow sun.

Scotch Broth is a thick, hearty soup perfect for chilly early-spring days, as it uses vegetables traditionally available at the end of winter.

2 pounds frozen lamb bones, no need
 to thaw
4 medium carrots, 1 quartered,
 3 coarsely chopped
1 medium onion, quartered
2 bay leaves
1 tablespoon black peppercorns
2 medium turnips, peeled and coarsely
 chopped

2 medium leeks, cleaned and coarsely
 chopped
¼ cup barley
3 tablespoons split peas
Salt
2 tablespoons chopped kale or fresh
 parsley (optional)

The day before serving, preheat the oven to 400°F. Line a roasting pan with aluminum foil, and roast the lamb bones for about 1 hour, or until thoroughly browned. Pour all the bones and juices into a kettle, draining the pan into the kettle to include all the browned-on bits—don't worry about separating out the fat; that will be done later. Add water to cover, the quartered carrot and onion, the bay leaves, and the peppercorns. Cover and bring to a boil over high heat; reduce the heat to low and simmer for 2 hours.

Strain the broth into a container. Separate the meat from the bones and add to the broth. Discard the remaining broth ingredients. Cool the broth mixture to room temperature and refrigerate overnight.

About 2 hours before serving time, take the broth from the refrigerator and remove the fat. Measure the congealed broth and combine in a large saucepan with enough water to make 3 quarts. Add the chopped carrots, turnips, and leeks, along with the barley, the split peas, and 1 teaspoon salt. Bring to a boil and simmer, covered, for about 1½ hours, or until the barley is tender. If desired, add the kale. Add salt if needed and serve.

Helen and Dan Flaherty decided that they wanted a farm where their two young sons could run freely. Their farm, Tir na nOg, in upstate New York, is a grass-based enterprise, and their eggs, chickens, beef, lamb, and pork products are distributed to high-end restaurants and CSAs throughout New York City.

ROASTED CHICKEN WITH SWISS CHARD AND FRESH CORN RELISH

MAKES 4 SERVINGS

2 tablespoons cider vinegar
2 tablespoons vegetable oil
1 tablespoon sugar
1 teaspoon chili powder
1 teaspoon ground cumin
Salt and freshly milled black pepper
1 cup fresh corn kernels

1 large red bell pepper, chopped
2 green onions, thinly sliced
2 (3-pound) organic chickens, halved
1 tablespoon chopped fresh thyme
1½ pounds Swiss chard, rinsed,
    drained, and thickly sliced

Combine the vinegar, oil, sugar, chili powder, cumin, and salt and pepper to taste in a bowl. Stir in the corn, bell pepper, and onions. Cover and refrigerate until ready to serve.

Preheat the oven to 400°F. Arrange the chicken halves in a large roasting pan. Sprinkle with the thyme, ½ teaspoon salt, and ¼ teaspoon pepper. Roast for 45 to 60 minutes, until the internal temperature reaches 180°F.

Meanwhile, simmer the greens in a large pot of boiling water until wilted. Drain well.

When the chicken is cooked through, move it to a plate or board; add the Swiss chard to the roasting pan and stir until the pan juices are combined with the greens. Taste and add salt, if necessary. Divide the Swiss chard among 4 plates; top each with a chicken half and serve with the corn relish.

GRILLED WILD ALASKAN HALIBUT

MAKES 4 SERVINGS

Brooke Williamson, executive chef of Zax restaurant in Los Angeles, contributed this easy-to-make halibut recipe. Brooke buys about 10 percent of her restaurant's produce from Coastal Organics, a nearby farm. She does so for environmental reasons, but she also believes that the freshness of flavor that local products provide is essential to good cooking. An added bonus: customers seem to like it. When she adds a delicious local heirloom tomato to a dish, she often encourages the staff to tell diners about it as they outline the menu. Says Brooke: "If you talk a little about a food's origin, it sparks interest in the customer's eye."

4 medium Yukon gold potatoes, scrubbed
Olive oil
4 fresh thyme sprigs
Salt and freshly milled black pepper
1 large eggplant, peeled and cut into ¾-inch cubes
1 large tomato, coarsely chopped
3 tablespoons sugar
4 garlic cloves
4 teaspoons sherry vinegar
1 teaspoon ground coriander
4 (6-ounce) halibut fillets
Herb Vinaigrette (recipe follows)

Preheat the oven to 350°F. Toss the whole potatoes with ¼ cup olive oil, the thyme, and salt and pepper to taste. Place in a roasting pan, cover with aluminum foil, and roast for about 45 minutes, or until the potatoes are soft.

Heat ½ cup olive oil in a large saucepan and add the eggplant, tomato, sugar, garlic, vinegar, and coriander. Cook on medium heat until the eggplant is soft, about 5 minutes. Season with salt and pepper to taste and set aside.

Rub the halibut with olive oil, and salt and pepper to taste, and grill on both sides to the desired temperature.

To serve, cut the potatoes in half and arrange on 4 plates. Top with the warm eggplant mixture and then the halibut. Drizzle the halibut and the plates with the herb vinaigrette.

HERB VINAIGRETTE: Whisk together ¼ cup olive oil, 2 tablespoons sherry vinegar, 1 tablespoon sugar, 1 tablespoon chopped garlic, 1 tablespoon chopped shallot, 1 tablespoon chopped fresh parsley, 1 teaspoon chopped fresh thyme, ¼ teaspoon chopped fresh rosemary, ¼ teaspoon chopped fresh mint, and salt and freshly milled black pepper to taste.

Cooking Meat

The single biggest error most people commit when cooking meat, especially grass-fed meats, is overcooking. Commercial meats, especially pork and turkey, are injected with saltwater solutions. This adds to the weight, so a greater profit is made, but it also lengthens cooking time and causes the meats to shrink noticeably. You will not find this to be the case with grass-fed meats. They are going to cook much faster than what you are used to, especially in the case of turkey. A rule of thumb is to expect the meat to cook in one-third to one-half less time than conventional meats. The easiest way to prevent overcooking is to use a good cooking thermometer—not a meat thermometer. A meat thermometer is not terribly accurate, and it is left in the meat while it cooks. A chef's thermometer has a small dial and is used to periodically check the internal temperature. I strongly prefer the digital thermometers (about $25), but the dial ones ($8 to $15) will work as well. You want to measure the temperature in the thickest part of the meat. In poultry, this will be the breast and/or thigh. Here is the most important part! Meat continues to cook even after it has been removed from the heat source; therefore, you want to stop cooking the meat just before it has reached the desired doneness. It will finish cooking on its own from the residual heat. Here are the recommended final temperatures for meats. I remove them from the heat source when they are 5 to 10 degrees below the desired temperature and allow them to finish cooking via residual heat.

Beef
Rare—120 degrees
Medium-rare—125 degrees
Medium—130 degrees
Medium-well—135 degrees
Well—140 degrees

Chicken and Turkey
160 degrees

Pork
150 degrees

—from Jenny Drake, Peaceful Pastures Farm, Hickman, Tennessee

VEAL POT ROAST

MAKES 6 SERVINGS

Sunnyside Farm in Nichols, New York, is a grass-based seasonal dairy run by Pam and Rob Moore. In addition to milk, the Moores produce other grass-fed products, such as raw-milk cheese, grass-fattened beef, suckling veal, milk-fed pork, and eggs. The farm and all its products are certified organic.

2 pounds veal London broil, arm, or
 chuck roast
3 to 4 cups buttermilk
2 tablespoons unsalted butter
2 tablespoons extra-virgin olive oil
1 large onion, cut into ½-inch wedges
½ cup red wine or additional stock

1½ cups stock (meat, poultry,
 or vegetable)
1 to 2 sprigs thyme, tied together,
 or about ½ teaspoon dried thyme
1 pound potatoes, small or cut up
½ pound carrots, cut up
Salt and freshly milled black pepper
Flour (optional)

Place veal roast in a nonreactive bowl and cover with buttermilk (see Note). Cover bowl and marinate veal in refrigerator overnight. Remove roast from buttermilk and pat dry.

Preheat oven to 300°F. Heat butter and olive oil in heavy Dutch oven; add the roast and brown it on all sides, about 8 minutes, adding the onion for the last 3 minutes. Remove the roast and pour off any excess fat.

Add wine, stock, and thyme to Dutch oven; bring mixture to a boil, stirring to loosen browned-on bits. Return roast to Dutch oven; cover and roast 2 to 2½ hours or until tender. Add potatoes and carrots when roast seems almost tender and cook for 20 minutes. Season to taste with salt and pepper. Remove roast and vegetables to serving platter.

If desired, thicken broth for gravy. Mix water into ¼ to ⅓ cup flour until it is the consistency of heavy cream. Whisk enough of the flour mixture into the boiling stock to thicken. Serve gravy with roast.

NOTE: If you don't have buttermilk, you can substitute plain milk mixed with 1 tablespoon vinegar, lemon juice, or kombucha tea per cup of milk.

RESOURCES

There are more than a thousand CSAs in the United States, and new ones form every year. If you're looking for a CSA in your area, the best source is the Robyn Van En Center for CSA Resources, a clearinghouse for information about Community Supported Agriculture all over the country. The center maintains the most complete list of CSAs, categorized by state. It also provides a history and explanation of the CSA movement and a list of links to related organizations.

Contact them at

Robyn Van En Center for CSA Resources
Fulton Center for Sustainable Living
Wilson College
1015 Philadelphia Ave.
Chambersburg, PA 17201
Phone: 717-264-4141, ext. 3352   Fax: 717-264-1578
e-mail: info@csacenter.org
http://www.csacenter.org

Here are some other organizations that list CSA information:

Biodynamic Farming and Gardening Association
P.O. Box 29135
Bldg. 1002B, Thoreau Center, The Presidio
San Francisco, CA 94129-0135
Phone: 888-516-7797   Fax: 415-561-7796
e-mail: biodynamic@aol.com
http://www.biodynamics.com

How to Find a CSA
Near You

Center for Agroecology and Sustainable Food Systems
University of California–Santa Cruz
http://zzyx.ucsc.edu/casfs/community/csap.html

Farmer's Market Online
Community Support (Resource Page)
http://www.farmersmarketonline.com

Local Harvest
A public service project of Ocean Group for CSAs and farmers' markets
http://www.localharvest.org

National Campaign for Sustainable Agriculture
P.O. Box 396
Pine Bush, NY 12566
Phone: 845-744-8448   Fax: 845-744-8477
e-mail: campaign@sustainableagriculture.net
http://www.sustainableagriculture.net

Organic Consumers Association
6114 Hwy. 61
Little Marais, MN 55614
Phone: 218-226-4164   Fax: 218-226-4157
e-mail: info@organicconsumers.org
http://www.purefood.org

The Small Farm Program
USDA Cooperative State Research, Education, and Extension Service
http://www.reeusda.gov/smallfarm

Small Farms
A component of the Cornell University Agriculture, Food and Communities
   website
http://www.cals.cornell.edu/agfoodcommunity/afc.cfm

Sustainable Agriculture Network
http://www.sare.org/

Urban Agriculture Notes/City Farmer
Canada's Office of Urban Agriculture
http://www.cityfarmer.org/

USDA Agricultural Marketing Service
Farmer Direct Marketing, Farm Direct Marketing Bibliography, Part 8
http://www.ams.usda.gov/directmarketing/b_8.htm

In Canada, the groups to contact are

Canadian Organic Growers
P.O. Box 6408, Station J
Ottawa, Ontario, K2A 3Y6 CANADA
Phone: 613-231-9047
e-mail: info@cog.ca
http://www.cog.ca/

Équiterre
2177, rue Masson, Bureau 317
Montreal, Quebec, H2H 1B1 CANADA
Phone: 514-522-2000   Fax: 514-522-1227
e-mail: ijoncas@equiterre.qc.ca
http://www.equiterre.qc.ca

Ecological Agriculture Projects
McGill University (Macdonald Campus)
Ste Anne-de-Bellevue, Quebec, H9X 3V9 CANADA
Phone: 514-398-7771   Fax: 514-398-7621
e-mail: info@eap.mcgill.ca
http://eap.mcgill.ca/

If you don't find a CSA near you on any of the lists maintained by these organizations, that doesn't mean there isn't one. Ask at your local cooperative extension office (they are usually in the phone book under Department of Agriculture) or ask farmers at the local farmers' market if they run a CSA. Call the nearest CSA farm (even if it is three hundred miles away) and ask if it knows of a farm that is closer to you. Most CSA farmers are happy to help their colleagues.

The following state and regional organizations maintain lists of newly formed and about-to-be-formed CSAs; they often help bring members and farmers together and help in the development of new farms and new CSAs

California Certified Organic Farmers
1115 Mission St.
Santa Cruz, CA 95060
Phone: 831-423-2263 (toll-free in state:
    888-423-CCOF)
Fax: 831-423-4528
http://www.ccof.org

Carolina Farm Stewardship Association
P.O. Box 448
Pittsboro, NC 27312
Phone: 919-542-2402
Fax: 919-542-7401
e-mail: cfsa@carolinafarmstewards.org

Center for Integrated Agricultural
    Systems
1450 Linden Dr., Room 146
University of Wisconsin
Madison, WI 53706
Phone: 608-265-3704
e-mail: jhendric@macc.wisc.edu

Community Alliance with Family
    Farmers
36355 Russell Blvd.
P.O. Box 363
Davis, CA 95617
Phone: 530-756-8518
Fax: 530-756-7857
http://www.caff.org

Community Food Security Coalition
P.O. Box 209
Venice, CA 90294
Phone/Fax: 310-822-5410
e-mail: asfisher@aol.com
http://www.foodsecurity.org

CSA Farm Network Publications
Steve Gilman
130 Ruckytucks Rd.
Stillwater, NY 12170
Phone: 518-583-4613
e-mail: sgilman@netheaven.com

CSA West
Center for Sustainable Food Systems
University of California–Santa Cruz
1156 High St.
Santa Cruz, CA 95064
Phone: 408-459-3964
Fax: 408-459-2799
e-mail: farmcsa@aol.com
http://www.caff.org/caff/programs/

Farming Alternatives Program
216 Warren Hall
Cornell University
Ithaca, NY 14853
Phone: 607-255-9832
e-mail: jmp32@cornell.edu
http://www.cals.cornell.edu/dept/ruralsoc/
    fap/fap.html

The Food and Farm Connection
P.O. Box 477
Dixon, NM 87527
Phone: 505-579-4386
http://www.foodfarm.wsu.edu

Future Harvest–Chesapeake Alliance for
    Sustainable Agriculture
P.O. Box 337
106 Market Ct.
Stevensville, MD 21666
Phone: 410-604-2681
Fax: 410-604-2689
e-mail: fhcasa@umail.umd.edu
http://www.futureharvestcasa.org/

Georgia Organics, Inc.
PMB 200
3895 Cherokee St. NW, Suite 200
Kennesaw, GA 30144-6727
Phone: 770-993-5534 or 608-873-8224
    (direct)
www.georgiaorganics.org

Great Lakes Area CSA Coalition
    (GLACSAC)
C/O Peter Seely
7065 Silver Spring Lane
Plymouth, WI 53073
Phone: 414-437-5971

Hartford Food System
509 Weathersfield Ave.
Hartford, CT 06114
Phone: 860-296-9325
e-mail: hn2838@handsnet.org

Iowa Network for Community
    Agriculture (INCA)
1465 120th St.
Kanawha, IA 50447
Phone: 515-495-6367
e-mail: libland@kalnet.com

Just Food/NYC Sustainable Food System
    Alliance
307 Seventh Ave., Suite 1201
New York, NY 10001
Phone: 212-645-9880
Fax: 212-645-9881
e-mail: info@justfood.org
http://www.justfood.org

Land Stewardship Project
2200 Fourth St.
White Bear Lake, MN 55110
Phone: 651-653-0618
Fax: 651-653-0589
e-mail: lspwbl@mtn.org
http://landstewardshipproject.org

Leopold Center for Sustainable
    Agriculture
209 Curtiss Hall
Iowa State University
Ames, IA 50011-1050
Phone: 515-294-3711
e-mail: leocenter@iastate.edu
http://www.leopold.iastate.edu

Madison Area Community Supported
    Agricultural Coalition (MACSAC)
4915 Monona Dr., Suite 304
Monona, WI 53716
Phone: 608-226-0300
Fax: 608-226-0301
e-mail: macsac@wrdc.org
http://www.wisc.edu/cias/macsac

Maine Organic Farmers and Gardeners
    Association
P.O. Box 2176
Augusta, ME 04338-2176
Phone: 207-622-3118
e-mail: mofga@mofga.org
http://www.mofga.org

Michael Fields Agricultural Institute
W2493 County Road East
East Troy, WI 53120
Phone: 414-642-3303
Fax: 414-642-4028
e-mail: mfai@mfai.org

Michigan Organic Food and Farm
  Alliance (MOFFA)
P.O. Box 530
Hartland, MI 48353-0530
Phone: 810-632-7952
Fax: 810-632-7620
e-mail: hnccinc@ismi.net
http://www.moffa.org

Minnesota Food Association
1916 Second Ave. South
Minneapolis, MN 55403-3927
Phone: 612-872-3298
http://www.misa.umn.edu/

Minnesota Institute for Sustainable
  Agriculture (MISA)
411 Borlaug Hall
University of Minnesota
Saint Paul, MN 55108-1013
Phone: 612-625-8235
Fax: 612-625-1268
e-mail: misamail@gold.tc.umn.edu
http://www.misa.umn.edu/csag.html

New England Small Farm Institute
P.O. Box 937
Belchertown, MA 01007
Phone: 413-323-4531
Fax: 413-323-9594
e-mail: info@smallfarm.org
http://www.smallfarm.org

New Mexico Farmers Marketing
  Association
Phone: 888-983-4400
e-mail: marketsnm@nets.com
http://www.farmersmarketsnm.org

Northeast Organic Farming Association
  (NOFA)
411 Sheldon Rd.
Barre, MA 01005
Phone: 978-355-2853
Fax: 978-355-4046
e-mail: jackkitt@aol.com
http://www.nofamass.org
(Also NOFA state chapters involved in
  CSA: New York, Vermont, New
  Hampshire, New Jersey, Connecticut)

Northeast Sustainable Agriculture
  Working Group (NESAWG)
P.O. Box 608
Belchertown, MA 01007-0608
Phone: 413-323-4531
Fax: 413-323-9595
e-mail: nesfi@igc.apc.org

Northern Plains Sustainable Agriculture
  Society
9824 Seventy-ninth St. SE
Fullerton, ND 58441-9725
Phone/Fax: 701-883-4304
e-mail: tpnpsas@drservices.com
http://www.npsas.org

Ohio Ecological Food and Farming
  Association
P.O. Box 82234
Columbus, OH 43202
Phone: 614-421-2022
Fax: 614-421-2011
http://www.oeffa.org

Oregon Tilth
1860 Hawthorne Ave. NE, Suite 200
Salem, OR 97303
Phone: 503-378-0690
Fax: 503-378-0809
e-mail: organic@tilth.org
http://www.tilth.org

Pennsylvania Association for Sustainable
   Agriculture
P.O. Box 419
Millheim, PA 16854
Phone: 814-349-9856
Fax: 814-349-9840
e-mail: info@pasafarming.org
http://www.pasafarming.org

Pennsylvania Certified Organic
1919 General Potter Hwy., Suite 1
Centre Hall, PA 16828
Phone: 814-364-1344
Fax: 814-364-4431
e-mail: paorganic@aol.com
http://www.hometown.aol.com/paorganic

Prairieland CSA
P.O. Box 1404
Champaign, IL 61824-1404
Phone: 217-239-3686
e-mail: abarnes@prairienet.org
http://www.prairienet.org/pcsa/pcsa.htm

Seattle Tilth Association
4649 Sunnyside Ave. North, Room 1
Seattle, WA 98103
Phone: 206-633-0451
e-mail: tilth@seattletilth.org
http://www.seattletilth.org

Small Farm Center
University of California–Davis
1 Shields Ave.
Davis, CA 95616-8699
Phone: 530-752-8136
Fax: 530-752-7716
http://www.sfc.ucdavis.edu

Southern Sustainable Agriculture
   Working Group/Community Farm
   Alliance
P.O. Box 324
Elkins, AR 72727-0324
Phone: 501-587-0888
Fax: 501-587-1333
e-mail: ssfarm@juno.com

Sustainable Earth, Inc.
100 Georgeton Ct.
West Lafayette, IN 47906
Phone: 765-463-9366
Fax: 765-497-0164
e-mail: sbonney@iquest.net

Texas Organic Growers Association
   (TOGA)
P.O. Box 15211
Austin, TX 78761
Phone: 877-326-5175
Fax: 512-842-1293
e-mail: suejefi@aol.com
http://www.texasorganicgrowers.org/

Wisconsin Rural Development Center
4915 Monona Dr., Suite 304
Monona, WI 53716
Phone: 608-226-0300
Fax: 608-226-0301

e-mail: wrdc@execpc.com
(Works with Madison Area Community
    Supported Agriculture Coalition
    [MACSAC])

PUBLICATIONS

There's a full list of CSA-related publication at the CASA Center website. Here are some from farms that participated in the creation of this book:

Sharing the Harvest
Elizabeth Henderson with Robyn Van En
(can be ordered on the CSA Center
    website)

From *Asparagus to Zucchini: A Guide to
    Farm-Fresh, Seasonal Produce*
Written by members of the Madison
    Area Community Supported
    Agriculture Coalition (MACSAC)
(can be ordered on the CSA Center
    website)

*ROOT: A Seasonal Journal from Mariquita
    Farm*
c/o Mariquita Farm
P.O. Box 2065
Watsonville, CA 95077
Subscribe through
    info@rootjournal.com

The Community Farm Newsletter
c/o Five Spring Farms
3480 Potter Rd.
Bear Lake, MI 49614
831-761-3226
csafarm@jackpine.com
fivespringsfarm.itgo.com

Organic Matters
Henry Brockman
available through TerraBooks:
    309-965-2407

How to Start a CSA

Finally, if you have determined that there is no CSA near you, if you think your area can support a farm through a CSA, or if you have a farm and would like to sell shares—consider starting one yourself. In some cases, the farmer takes on the burden of finding members and making all the decisions about pricing, what's in a share, how the shares are delivered. In some cases, the farmers even deliver right to the members' doors. Many CSAs are run with the help of their members. A few members who are willing to take on more responsibility (they're usually called the core group) meet with the farmer to decide how many members are needed, how much to charge, how to let the farmer know what the members like and dislike. In some cases, members volunteer (or are required to volunteer) to recruit new members, to collect membership fees, to help run the distribution centers, and to work on the farm (which for some members is one of the great benefits of joining).

Running a CSA requires a great deal of work and flexibility for both members and farmers; CSAs are great, but they are not easy. Farmers receive money up front, when they need it for seed and equipment, and are guaranteed that their entire crop will be sold—but they have to plant a full range of produce, not just a few crops that they like best; they have to give up some autonomy (sometimes just a bit, sometimes quite a lot, depending on the agreement between farmer and members). And members receive fresher, better produce than they would find elsewhere, usually at lower prices; and they enjoy a priceless connection to their food source and the knowledge that they are helping to sustain the local agriculture. But they accept the risk of a poor harvest and agree to accept whatever the farmer harvests, so they can't demand out-of-season vegetables, fruits that can't be grown in their area, or a crop that has failed due to weather or other conditions.

So don't start a CSA without knowing the difficulties and problems that can arise. Talk to other people who are involved, study all the information from the Internet, join another CSA for a season (even if it is far away) so you can experience it firsthand. And farmers and members should fully discuss all the issues that may confront them so that expectations are clear on both sides. Don't go in blind—but don't be discouraged by the difficulty either, because thousands of CSAs are operating successfully and happily all over the country.

ISSUES

Most people who are interested in Community Supported Agriculture are also interested in food issues that, in the opinion of some experts, have become dangerous crises. Environmentalists and farm activists fear that current farming practices endanger our water supply, our health, and the growth and development of future generations. Here are some websites that discuss these issues:

Sustainable Agriculture

Many large commercial farms employ methods that might make food cheaper today—but these practices will eventually deplete the environment of natural resources and create an atmosphere where nothing can grow. Most CSA farms farm sustainably. A definition of sustainable agriculture, from the U.S. Department of Agriculture (USDA) Sustainable Agriculture Research and Education (SARE) program:

> Sustainable agriculture refers to an agricultural production and distribution system that

- achieves the integration of natural biological cycles and controls
- protects and renews soil fertility and the natural resource base
- optimizes the management and use of on-farm resources
- reduces the use of nonrenewable resources and purchased production inputs
- provides an adequate and dependable farm income
- promotes opportunity in family farming and farm communities
- minimizes adverse impacts on health, safety, wildlife, water quality, and the environment

For more information about sustainable agriculture:

Center for a Livable Future at Johns Hopkins School of Public Health
http://www.jhsph.edu/environment/

Land Stewardship Project
http://www.landstewardshipproject.org/

National Campaign for Sustainable Agriculture
http://www.sustainableagriculture.net/

USDA Sustainable Agriculture Research and Education Program
http://www.sare.org/

Genetic Modifications

Scientific advances have made it possible for breeders to alter the genetic composition of plants. This sounds wonderful, and maybe it is; but have we done enough research? The possibilities and dangers are discussed on the following websites:

Sierra Club
http://www.sierraclub.org/biotech/references.asp

Union of Concerned Scientists
http://www.ucsusa.org/index.html

Clean Water and Pesticides

Agricultural runoff is a major cause of pollution in our environment. The issue is discussed on the following websites:

Beyond Pesticides
http://www.beyondpesticides.org/main.html

Sierra Club
http://www.sierraclub.org/factoryfarms/factsheets

Food Additives

Most livestock farms that serve the CSA community avoid the use of antibiotics and hormones that have promoted antibiotic-resistant strains of viruses and other health problems. This website focuses on the safety of food additives:

Alliance for the Prudent Use of Antibiotics
http://nutrition.tufts.edu/programs/afe/

Organic Standards

In October 2002, after years of discussion and controversy, the USDA Organic Standards Act became law. Many organic consumers and farmers are pleased that the word "organic" has a meaning. Others are worried that the organic standards are not stringent enough and that the new standards favor large farms over small. In fact, a group of small farms have banded together to meet the needs of small farmers that might be harmed by the new laws. The following websites discuss the issue from several standpoints. The first item in this section is the website for Certified Naturally Grown, the organization formed to meet the needs of smaller farmers.

Certified Naturally Grown
http://www.naturallygrown.org/press.html

Maine Organic Farmers and Gardeners Association
http://www.mofga.org

USDA National Organics Standards Program
http://www.ams.usda.gov/nop/

Antiorganic Attacks

In the past few years, several articles have appeared in the press that attack the organic industry, casting doubt on its value and in some cases even on its safety. Their claims have been fully countered and shown to be false; if you'd like to hear the full story, please see the following website: http://www.vegsource.com/articles/organics.2020.htm

The Corporatization of Farming

The issue that CSA most directly addresses is the destruction of family farms, the transfer of control of our food systems from individuals to corporations. Family Farmer is an organization that supports the family farmer; see its website for information about why we want to stop the corporatization of farming:

http://www.familyfarmer.org

Contributing Farms

ALABAMA
Mount Laurel Organic Gardens
Jerry Spencer
1185 Dunavant Valley Rd.
Birmingham, AL 35242
Phone/Fax: 205-991-0042
mtlaurelorganics@aol.com
http://www.mtlaurelorganics.com
Birmingham

ALASKA
Calypso Farm and Ecology Center
Tom Zimmer and Susan Willsrud
P.O. Box 106
Ester, AK 99725
Phone: 907-451-0691
tom@calypsofarm.org
http://www.calypsofarm.org
Ester and Fairbanks

ARIZONA
Double Check Ranch
Jean Schwennesen
69970 E. Freeman Rd.
Winkelman, AZ 85292
Phone: 520-357-6515
Schwennesen@juno.com
http://www.greatbeef.com
Tucson Area

CALIFORNIA
Eatwell Farm
Frances and Nigel Walker
9420 Stevenson Bridge Rd.
Winters, CA 95694
Phone: 800-648-9894 or 530-759-8221
office@eatwell.com
http://www.eatwell.com
San Francisco, Berkeley, Oakland,
    San Rafael, Davis

Fairview Gardens
Michael Ableman
598 N. Fairview Ave.
Goleta, CA 93117
Phone: 805-967-7369
Fax: 805-967-0188
fairviewg@aol.com
http://www.fairviewgardens.org
Santa Barbara, Goleta, Montecito

Farm Fresh to You
Kathleen Barsotti
23808 State Hwy. 16
Capay, CA 95607
Phone: 800-796-6009
Fax: 530-796-3344
office@farmfreshtoyou.com
http://www.farmfreshtoyou.com/
East Bay, Marin County, San Francisco,
    and the Bay Peninsula

Flora Bella Farm
James and Bettina Birch
P.O. Box 271
Three Rivers, CA 93271
Phone: 559-561-3613
brchfarm@inreach.com
Three Rivers

Full Circle Organic Farm
Marcie Rosenzweig
3377 Early Times Lane
Auburn, CA 95603
Phone: 530-885-9201
fullcircle@jps.net
Central and South Placer County

Huasna Valley Farm
Ron and Jenn Skinner
5420 Huasna Townsite Rd.
Arroyo Grande, CA 93420
Phone/Fax: 805-473-3827
huasna@tcsn.net
San Luis Obispo County

Laguna Farms
Scott Mathieson
1764 Cooper Rd.
Sebastopol, CA 95472
Phone: 707-823-0823
organic@metro.net
http://www.lagunafarm.com
Sebastopol, Santa Rosa, Petaluma

Live Earth Farm
Thomas Broz
172 Litchfield Lane
Watsonville, CA 95076
Phone: 831-763-2448
info@liveearthfarm.com
http://www.liveearthfarm.com/
Monterey Bay and San Francisco Bay
   Areas

Mariquita Farms
Julia Wiley
P.O. Box 2065
Watsonville, CA 95077
Phone: 831-761-3226
csa@mariquita.com
http://www.mariquita.com
Santa Cruz County and Silicon Valley

Seabreeze Organic Farm
Stephenie Caughlin
3909 Arroyo Sorrento Rd.
San Diego, CA 92130
Phone: 858-481-0209
Fax: 858-481-4914
Seabreezeorganic@sbcglobal.net
http://www.seabreezed.com
San Diego County

Tierra Miguel Foundation CSA
Robert Farmer
P.O. Box 1065
Pauma Valley, CA 92061
Phone: 760-742-1151 or 760-742-1199
Fax: 769-742-1151
csa@tierramiguel.org
http://www.tierramiguel.org
San Diego County, Orange County,
   Los Angeles County

Winter Creek Gardens
Nina Andres and Chelsea Becker
P.O. Box 31
Rumsey, CA 95679
Phone: 530-796-2243
csa@wintercreekgardens.com
http://www.wintercreekgardens.com
San Francisco Bay Area, Sacramento,
   Marin, Davis

CONNECTICUT
White Gate Farm
Pauline Lord and David Harlow
83 Upper Pattagansett Rd.
P.O. Box 250
East Lyme, CT 06333
Phone: 860-739-2728
paulinelord@earthlink.net
Old Saybrook, Old Lyme, East Lyme,
   New London

FLORIDA
Sweetwater Organic Community Farm
Rick Martinez
6942 West Comanche Ave.
Tampa, FL 33634
Phone: 813-887-4066
Fax: 813-889-8218
rickinsp@aol.com
http://www.sweetwater-organic.org
Tampa Bay Area

GEORGIA
Boann's Banks Farms
Chris and Eric Wagoner
310 Woody Road
Royston, GA 30662
Phone: 706-245-9774
csa@boannsbanks.com
http://www.boannsbanks.com
Athens and Clarke, Madison, Franklin,
   Oconee, and Oglethorpe Counties

ILLINOIS
Angelic Organics
John Peterson and Bob Bower
1547 Rockton Rd.
Caledonia, IL 61011
Phone: 815-389-2746
Fax: 815-389-3106
CSA@AngelicOrganics.com
http://www.angelic-organics.com/
Northern Illinois

Henry's Farm
Terra Brockman
1569 Sugar Hill Lane
Congerville, IL 61729
Phone: 309-965-2407
terrabooks@earthlink.net
http://www.henrysfarm.com
Bloomington and Peoria

IOWA
Local Harvest CSA
Susan Zacharakis-Jutz
5025 120th St. NE
Solon, IA 52333
Phone: 319-644-3052
zjfarm@ia.net
Iowa City, Cedar Rapids, and
   surrounding counties

Sunflower Fields Family Farm and CSA
Linda and Michael Nash
776 Old Stage rd.
Postville, IA 52162
Phone: 319-864-3847 or 888-571-5472
Fax: 319-864-3837
sunspot@netins.net
http://www.sunflower-fields.com
Northeast Iowa, including Allamakee,
    Clayton, and Fayette

KANSAS
Full Circle Farm
Katherine Kelly and Carol Burns
4223 Gibbs Rd.
P.O. Box 6043
Kansas City, KS 66106
Phone: 913-515-2426
fullcirclefarm@msn.com
http://www.fullcirclefarmkc.com
Metro Kansas City

KENTUCKY
Bugtussle Organic Farm
Eric and Cher Smith
750 Rack Creek Rd.
Gamaliel, KY 42140
Phone: 270-427-8315
bugtussleorganicfarm@hotmail.com
Nashville

Dogwood Spring Organic Farm
Chris and Christy Korrow
2000 Bullridge Rd.
Burkesville, KY 42717
Phone: 270-864-4167
dogwoodspring@accessky.net
http://theruralcenter.org
Nashville

Hill and Hollow CSA
Robin Verson and Paul Bela
8707 Breeding Rd.
Edmonton, KY 42129
Phone: 270-432-0567
hhcsa@scrtc.com
Nashville

MAINE
Sunrise Acres Farm
Sally Merrill
42 Winn Rd.
Cumberland, ME 04021
sam082400@aol.com
Portland

MARYLAND
From the Ground Up
Carrie Cochran
Clagett Farm
11904 Old Marlboro Pike
Upper Marlboro, MD 20772
Phone: 301-627-4662
Fax: 301-574-3705
clagettfarm@cbf.org
http://www.clagettfarm.org/
Upper Marlboro, MD, and Anacostia
    and Southeastern D.C.

MASSACHUSETTS
Brookfield Farm CSA
Dan Kaplan
24 Hulst Rd.
South Amherst, MA 01002
Phone: 413-253-7991
bfcsa@aol.com

The Food Project
Don Zasada
P.O. Box 705
Lincoln, MA 01773
Phone: 781-259-8621
Fax: 781-259-9659
grower@thefoodproject.org
http://www.thefoodproject.org
Boston and Metro-West Suburbs,
   Middlesex County

Green Market Farm
John and Karen Wallman
710 Daniel Shays Hwy.
New Salem, MA 01355
Phone: 978-544-7911
Fax: 978-544-7587
greenmrkt@aol.com
http://www.HarvestAndHome.com
Central and Western Massachusetts

Many Hands Organic Farm
Julie Rawson, Jack Kittredge, and Dan
   Kittredge
411 Sheldon Rd.
Barre, MA 01005
Phone: 978-355-2853 or 978-355-2270
Fax: 978-355-4046
jackkitt@aol.com
Barre Area to Worcester, Gardam,
   Lemander, Athol

Marblehead Eco-Farm/Direct Co-op
Sara Lincoln-Harris
27 Gregory St.
Marblehead, MA 01945
Phone: 781-631-7214

Natural Roots Organic Farm
David Fisher
888 Shelburne Falls Rd.
Conway, MA 01341
Phone: 413-369-4269
Fax: 413-369-4299
Conway, Ashfield, Shelburne, Deerfield

MICHIGAN

Five Springs Farm CSA
Jo Meller and Jim Sluyter
3480 Potter Road
Bear Lake, MI 49614
Phone: 231-889-3216
csafarm@jackpine.com
http://tcf.itgo.com
Manistee, Benzie, Mason Counties in
   Northwestern Lower Michigan

Rocky Gardens
John and Diane Franklin
9635 Ryella Lane
Davisburg, MI 48350
Phone: 248-634-2291
Fax: 248-634-2251
diane@homeandgardensite.com
http://www.rockygardens.com
Oakland, Livingston, Genesee, and
   surrounding counties

MINNESOTA

Shaltz Farm
Zack and Holly Shaltz
05797 Lee Rd.
P.O. Box 136
Boyne City, MI 49712
Phone: 231-582-3206
zack@shaltzfarm.com or
   holly@shaltzfarm.com
http://www.shaltzfarm.com/

MISSOURI

Autumn Lane Farm
Roger, Brian, and Marilyn Ison
3487 N. Farm Rd. 127
Springfield, MO 65803
Phone: 417-833-2072
autumnln@dialus.com
Greater Springfield, Greene, and
    Christian Counties

MONTANA

Gaia Gardens
Brad and Kim Bauerly
6227 Forswall Rd.
Belgrade, MT 59714
Phone: 406-580-5785 or 406-580-5786
gaiagardens@theglobal.net
Bozeman and Gallatin and Park
    Counties

NEW HAMPSHIRE

Grande Hill Farm
Maria Southworth
81 Perkins Rd.
Madbury, NH 03820
Phone: 603-743-0093
MWSouthworth@attbi.com
Durham/Lee/Madbury in Strafford
    County (seacoast of NH)

NEW JERSEY

Cook College Student Organic Farm
    CSA
Ralph Coolman
69 Lipman Dr.
Rutgers University
New Brunswick, NJ 08903
Phone: 732-932-8406
Fax: 732-932-6837
coolman@aesop.rutgers.edu
http://aesop.rutgers.edu/~njuep/

The Philly Chile Company Farm CSA
Rob Ferber and Amanda McCutcheon
235 Swedesboro Rd.
Monroeville, NJ 08343
Phone: 856-358-1431
Fax: 856-358-1635
CSA@phillychile.com
http://www.phillychile.com
Salem, Gloucester, and Cumberland
    Counties, NJ; Philadelphia, PA

NEW MEXICO

The Rhubarb Ranch
Tom Hayden and Robyn Harrison
916 Allen Ct.
Socorro, NM 87801
Phone: 505-835-2542
robynj@nmt.edu
Socorro County

NEW YORK

Ash Grove Community Farm
Dori Green
1297 Martin Hill Rd.
Corning, NY 14830
Phone: 607-524-6741
dorigreen00@hotmail.com
http://www.ic.org/agrove
Corning and Elmira in Steuben County;
    Rochester, Syracuse, Buffalo

Canticle Farm (Allegany Agriculture)
Anne Rothmeier, OSF; Mark Printz
115 E. Main St.
Allegany, NY 14706
Phone: 716-373-1215 or 716-368-9714
    (cell)
arothmeier@earthlink.net
http://www.fsalleg.org/canticlefarm.htm
Allegany, Olean, Hinsdale, Portville,
    Cattaraugus County

Cooke Hollow Farm
Thomas Christenfeld
209 Cooke Hollow Rd.
Valley Falls, NY 12185
Phone: 518-692-9065
Fax: 518-692-8712
allegedfarm@post.harvard.edu
Brooklyn, Albany, Easton, Cambridge,
    Salem, Greenwich

Four Winds Farm
Jay and Polly Armour
158 Marabac Rd.
Gardiner, NY 12525
Phone: 845-255-3088
parmour255@aol.com
http://www.bestweb.net/~fourwind/

Genesee Valley Organic CSA
Elizabeth Henderson
2218 Welcher Rd.
Newark, NY 14513
Phone: 315-331-9029
Fax: 315-365-3299
ehendrsn@redsuspenders.com
http://www.gvocsa.org/

Grindstone Farm
Dick de Graff
780 Tinker Tavern Rd.
County Rt. 28
Pulaski, NY 13142
Phone: 315-298-4139
gsforganic@aol.com
http://www.grindstonefarm.com
Syracuse

Mountain Melody Gardens
Donna Karch
Rt. 23A
P.O. Box 75
Palenville, NY 12463
Phone: 518-678-9247

Narrow Bridge Farm
Jon Thorne and Tali Adini
P.O. Box 6766
Ithaca, NY 14851
Phone: 607-266-8464
talyon@juno.com
http://narrowbridgefarm.tripod.com/
Ithaca and Tompkins County

Ryder Farm
Katharine and Hall Gibson
404 Starr Ridge Rd.
Brewster, NY 10509
Phone: 914-279-3984
Southeastern Brewster County

Stoneledge Farm
Pete and Deborah Kavakos
359 Ross Ruland Rd.
South Cairo, NY 12482
Phone: 518-622-3003 or 212-502-8562
stoneledge@surferz.net
Upper East Side of Manhattan and
    Greene County

Tir na nOg Farm
Helen and Dan Flaherty
Walton, NY 13856
Phone: 607-865-8414

Whistle-Stop Gardens
Stuart McCarty
P.O. Box 70
Tunnel, NY 13848
Phone: 607-693-3378
Fax: 607-693-4415
whistop@ny.tds.net

Wood Creek Herb Farm
Brenda and Mike Henry
3995 Wood Creek Rd.
Rome, NY 13440
Phone: 315-339-1109
WOODCREEKFARM@cs.com
Rome, Utica, Oneida

NORTH CAROLINA
Mountain Harvest Organics
Julie Mansfield and Carl Evans
77 Wyatt Lane
Hot Springs, NC 28743-7715
Phone: 828-622-3654
farmer@MountainHarvestOrganic.com
http://www.MountainHarvestOrganic.
   com
Waynesville and Haywood County

Doubletree Farm
Cathy and Andy Bennett
835 Cargile Branch Rd.
Marshall, NC 28753
Phone: 828-689-3812
Marshall, Mars Hill, Weaverville,
   North Asheville

OHIO
Bluebird Hills Farm
Tim and Laurel Shouvlin
1243 Ryan Rd.
Farm address: 3617 Derr Rd.
Springfield, OH 45503
Phone/Fax: 937-390-6127
bluebirdhills@voyager.net
http://www.bluebirdhills.com
Springfield, Yellow Springs, Dayton,
   Beavercreek, Centerville

Boulder Belt Gardens CSA
Lucy and Eugene Goodman
4526 Crubaugh Rd.
New Paris, OH 45347
Phone: 937-273-3502
goodows@excite.com
http://www.angelfire.com/oh2/
   boulderbeltcsa/
Oxford and Preble County, OH;
   Richmond, IN; Wayne and Union City
   Counties, IN

Earth Source Organics
Leslie Markworth, Matt Tomaszewski,
   and Eric Pawlowski
P.O. Box 281
Batavia, OH 45103
Phone: 513-471-0755
lesmark73@aol.com
Greater Cincinnati and Northern
   Kentucky

Far Corner Farm CSA
Elise McMath and Kevin Smyth
12788 New England Rd.
Amesville, OH 45711
Phone: 740-448-2228
ab210@seorf.ohiou.edu
Columbus

OREGON

Dancin' Roots Farm
Shari Sirkin
74 NE Saratoga St.
Portland, OR 97211
Portland Metro Area

Denison Farms
Tom Denison
1835 Steele Ave.
Corvallis, OR 97330
Phone/Fax: 541-752-4156
denisont@peak.org
http://www.peak.org/~denisont
Portland, Salem, Eugene–Willamette
    Valley

Sauvie Island Organics
Shari Raider
20233 NW Sauvie Island Rd.
Portland, OR 97231
Phone: 503-621-6921
siorganics@aol.com
Portland Metro Area

PENNSYLVANIA

Common Ground Organic Farm
Leslie Zuck
RD #1, Box 151A
Spring Mills, PA 16875
Phone: 814-364-1344
Fax: 814-364-2330
CommonGro@aol.com
http://www.CommongroundFarm.com
Centre County

TENNESSEE

Peaceful Pastures
Jenny Drake
69 Cowan Valley Lane
Hickman, TN 38578
Phone: 615-683-4291
Fax: 615-683-5559
naturalmeat@aol.com
http://www.peacefulpastures.com
Nashville, Murfreesboro, Cookeville
    (ships nationwide)

TEXAS

Oasis Gardens CSA
Bill Enkhausen
7651 Delwau Lane
Austin, TX 78725
Phone: 512-386-7636 (Farmer Bill
    Enkhausen) or 512-288-3456 (Peter
    Fleury)
selwyn@austintx.com
http://www.greenbuilder.com/
    oasisgardenscsa/
Austin and Travis County

UTAH

Ranui Gardens
John Garofalo and Steve Erickson
1459 S. Hoytsville Rd.
Hoytsville, UT 84017
Phone: 435-336-2813 or 435-783-5908
Fax: 435-336-2331
ranui@allwest.net
http://www.ranui.com
Summit County

VERMONT

Clay Brook Farm
Bob Hill and Laury Shea
91 Old Pump Rd.
Jericho, VT 05465
Phone: 802-899-3743
Fax: 802-899-4774
boblaury@aol.com
Chittenden County

Urban Roots Farm
Jonathan Rappe
P.O. Box 5013
Burlington, VT 05401
Phone: 802-862-5929
jonathanrappe@cs.com
http://www.urbanrootsfarm.com
Greater Burlington Area

VIRGINIA

Bull Run Mountain Organic Farm
Leigh Hauter
4360 Highpoint Lane
The Plains, VA 20198
Phone: 703-754-4005
lh@pressroom.com
http://www.bullrunfarm.com/
Washington, D.C., and Northern
    Virginia

WASHINGTON

Full Circle Farm
Andrew Stout
P.O. Box 1178
North Bend, WA 98045
Phone: 425-831-2125
Fax: 425-831-2416
fcorganics@earthlink.net
Seattle Metro Area

Molly's Island Garden
Molly Petersons
3340 E. Craw Rd.
Langley, WA 98260
Phone: 360-321-5547
Fax: 360-321-5926
petersns@whidbey.com
South and Central Whidbey Island

Penn Cove Organics
Ulrike and Wendi Hilborn
1240 Arnold Rd.
Oak Harbor, WA 98277
Phone: 360-240-8125 or 360-661-1932
Fax: 360-240-8475
hilborn@whidbey.net
Whidbey Island: Oak Harbor,
    Coupeville, Freeland to Langley and
    Clinton; North Island; South Island;
    Seattle

The Wild Iris Farm
Nigel Day and Judith Caporiccio
579 S. Fortieth Ave.
West Richland, WA 99353
Phone: 509-967-2235 or 509-967-9485
Fax: 509-967-9485
wirisfarm@aol.com
Tri-Cities of the Mid-Columbia River
    Valley

WISCONSIN

Blackberry Hills Farm
Tim Hermann
E7339 County Rd. South
Wheeler, WI 54772
Phone: 715-658-1042
Menominee and Eau Claire County, WI,
    and Twin Cities, MN

Safe Home Farm
Robin Timm
9474 Greenwood Rd.
Platteville, WI 53818
Phone: 608-348-9827
jdrt@mhtc.net
Grant and Iowa County

Chefs Collaborative Members Who Contributed Recipes

Vince Alberici, Executive Chef
The Marker Restaurant
City Avenue and Marker Rd.
Philadelphia, PA
215-581-5000

Rick Bayless, Chef/Co-Owner
Frontera Grill/Topolobampo
445 N. Clark St.
Chicago, IL 60610
312-661-1434
http://www.fronterakitchens.com

Christopher Blobaum
Surf and Sand Resort
1555 South Coast Hwy.
Laguna Beach, CA 92651
800-664-7873

Shelley Boris, Executive Chef
Bill Brown's Restaurant and Bar
Garrison Golf Club
Garrison, NY 10525
845-424-3604
http://www.garrisongolfclub.com

Ross Browne, Executive Chef
Absinthe Brasserie and Bar
398 Hayes St.
San Francisco, CA 94102
415-551-1590

Suzanne Butler, Manager
Skagit Valley Farmers Market
P.O. Box 2053
Mount Vernon, WA 98274
360-336-0163

Rosemary and Fabrizio Chiariello
Gateway Inn and Restaurant
51 Walker St.
Lenox, MA 01240
413-637-2532 or 413-822-9488

Richard and Mary Anne Erickson,
    Chef/Owners
Blue Mountain Bistro
1633 Glasco Turnpike
Woodstock, NY 12498
914-679-8519

Jim and Ellen Gist
River Run Farm
19224 Swedetown Rd.
Clatskanie, OR 97016
503-728-4561
http://www.riverrunfarm.com

Reuben Haag, Executive Chef
Bon Appétit at Hamilton College
198 College Hill Rd.
Clinton, NY 13323
(not open to public)

Christopher Hastings
Hot and Hot Fish Club
2180 Eleventh Court South
Birmingham, AL 35205
205-933-5474
http://www.hotandhotfishclub.com

Judith Hausman
The Journal News
White Plains, NY 10604

Peter Hoffman, Chef/Owner
Savoy
70 Prince St.
New York, NY 10012-3306
212-219-8570

Roxanne Klein, Chef/Owner
Roxanne's
320 Magnolia Ave.
Larkspur, CA 94939
415-924-5004
http://www.roxraw.com

Michael Leviton, Chef/Co-Owner
Lumière
1293 Washington St.
West Newton, MA 02465
617-244-9199
http://www.lumiererestaurant.com

Waldy Malouf, Chef/Owner
Beacon Restaurant
25 W. Fifty-sixth St.
New York, NY 10019
212-332-0500
http://www.beaconnyc.com

John McReynolds, Chef
Café La Haye
140 E. Napa St.
Sonoma, CA 95476
707-935-9481
http://www.cafelahaye.com

Jeff Nagel, Chef
Caprine Estates, Willow Run Dairy
3669 Centerville Rd.
Bellbrook, OH 45305
937-848-7406

Ric Orlando
New World Home Cooking
Rt. 212
Saugerties, NY 12477
845-246-0900

Mardee Palacios, Sales and Marketing
    for Chef Miki Knowles
B&W Quality Growers
17825 79th St.
Fellsmere, FL 32948
772-571-0800
http://www.watercress.com

Lou Rook, Chef
Annie Gunn's
16806 Chesterfield Airport Rd.
Chesterfield, MO 63005
636-532-7684

Ben Schulman, Chef
Exxon Mobil headquarters
800 Bell St.
Houston, TX 77002

Bev Shaffer, Cooking School Director
Mustard Seed Market and Café
3888 West Market St.
Akron, OH 44333
330-666-7333
and
6025 Kruse Dr.
Solon, OH
440-519-3663
http://www.mustardseedmarket.com

Eileen and Gene Theil
Wholesale Organic Potatoes
P.O. Box 549
Joseph, OR 97846
541-432-2361
http://www.potatoman@eoni.com

Kevin von Klause, Executive
    Chef/Partner
White Dog Café
3420 Sansom St.
Philadelphia, PA 19104
215-386-9224
http://www.whitedog.com

Christine Wansleben, Chef, and Valeria
    Flynn, Chef
A Sharper Palate Catering Company
5511 Lakeside Ave.
Richmond, VA 23228
804-553-0495

Ronna N. Welsh, Sous-Chef
Danal Restaurant
90 E. Tenth St.
New York, NY 10003-ß5463
212-982-6930

Brooke Williamson
Zax Restaurant
11604 San Vicente Blvd.
Los Angeles, CA 90049
310-571-3800

INDEX

ABOUT THE AUTHORS

JOANNE LAMB HAYES has developed, tested, and written recipes for thirty-seven years. She is the author of *Grandma's Wartime Kitchen,* the coauthor of seven cookbooks, the former food editor of *Country Living Magazine,* and has worked in the test kitchens of *McCall's* and *Family Circle* magazines. She is a member of the Carnegie Hill/Yorkville CSA in Manhattan.

LORI STEIN is president of Layla Productions, a book production company that has completed more than two hundred books, including *Good Housekeeping's Recipe Collections* and *The American Garden Guides.* She is a member of the Carnegie Hill/Yorkville CSA and works with citywide CSA organizations in Manhattan.

Acknowledgments

To Gryphon Books, for their commitment, patience, and professionalism in digging up reference books for me on the 19th-century English banking system. Many thanks—you've spared me more sleepless nights than I can count.

To my family, the true-to-life embodiment of what Anastasia and Breanna's grandfather believed family ought to be. I love you.

THE GOLD COIN

To family—those special people
whose hearts and lives
are tied to yours.

Prologue

<figure>❧</figure>

Kent, England
August 1803

*T*hey made the pact when they were six.

They hadn't planned on making it. But drastic circumstances required drastic actions. And drastic circumstances were precisely what they found themselves in on that fateful night.

Fearfully, the two little girls hesitated at the doorway.

Crackling tension permeated the dining room. They peeked inside, freezing in their tracks as angry voices assailed them. They scooted backward, pressing themselves flat against the wall so as not to be spied.

"What the hell is wrong with discussing profits?" Lord George Colby barked, his sharp words hurled at his brother. "The fact that our business is making a fortune should please you as much as it does me."

"Tonight is not about profits, George," Lord Henry reminded him in a voice that was taut with repressed ire. "It's about family."

"Family? As in brotherly devotion?" A mocking laugh. "Don't insult me, Henry. The business is the only meaningful thing you and I share."

"You're right. More and more right every day. And I'm getting damned tired of trying to change that."

"Well, so much for sentiment," George noted scornfully. "And so much for this whole sham of a reunion."

"It wasn't meant to be a reunion." Clearly, Henry was striving for control. "It's Father's sixtieth birthday celebration. Or had you forgotten?"

"I've forgotten nothing. *Nothing.* Have you?"

The pointed barb sank in, blanketing the room in silence.

"They're fighting loud," Anastasia hissed, inching farther away from the doorway, and shoving one unruly auburn tress off her face. "Especially Uncle George. We're in trouble. *Big* trouble."

"I know." Her cousin Breanna gazed down at herself, her delicate features screwed up in distress as she surveyed her soiled party frock—which was identical to Anastasia's, only much filthier. "Father sounds really mad. And if he sees I got all dirty . . . and ruined the dress Grandfather gave me . . ." She began rubbing furiously at the mud and grass stains, pausing only to wipe streaks of dirt from her forearms.

Anastasia watched, chewing her lip, knowing this whole disaster was her fault. She'd been the one who insisted they sneak out of Medford Manor to play while the grown-ups talked. Now she wished she'd never suggested it. In fact, she wished it had been she, rather than Breanna, who had fallen into the puddle outside. Her father would have forgiven her. He was gentle and kind—well, at least when it came to her. When it came to almost everyone, in fact. Except for one person: his brother. He and Uncle George, though twins, were practically enemies.

Maybe that was because they were so different—except for their looks, which were identical, right down to their vivid coloring: jade green eyes and thick cinnamon hair, both of which she and Breanna had inherited. But in every other way their fathers were like day and night. Her own father had a quick mind and an easy nature. He embraced life, creative business ventures, and his family, while Uncle George was stiff in manner, rigid in expectations, and downright intimidating when crossed.

Especially when the one who crossed him was his daughter.

"Stacie!" Breanna's frantic hiss yanked Anastasia out of her reverie. "What should I do?"

Anastasia was used to being the one whose ideas got them both in and out of trouble. But this time the trouble they'd be facing was bad. And the person who'd be paying the price would be Breanna. Well, that was something Anastasia couldn't—*wouldn't*—allow.

Her mind began racing, seeking ways to keep Uncle George from seeing Breanna—or at least from seeing her frock.

Absently, Anastasia studied her own party dress, noting that other than a fine layer of dirt along the hem, it was respectably clean.

Now *that* spawned an idea.

"I know! We can change dresses." Even as she spoke, she spied Wells, the Medford butler, striding down the endless corridor, heading in their direction. Any second he would spot them—if he hadn't done so already. It was too late for scrambling in and out of their dresses.

"No," she amended dejectedly. "We don't have time. It would've worked, too, 'cause our dresses look exactly the same—" Abruptly she broke off, her eyes lighting up as she contemplated another, far better and more intriguing possibility. "So do we."

Breanna's brows drew together. "So do we . . . what?"

"Look exactly the same. Everyone says so. Our fathers are twins. Our mothers are sisters—or at least they were until yours went to heaven. No one can ever tell us apart. Even Mama and Papa get confused sometimes. So why don't you be me and I'll be you?"

"You mean switch places?" Breanna's fear was supplanted by interest. "Can we do that?"

"Why not?" Swiftly, Anastasia combed her fingers through her tangled masses of coppery hair, trying—with customary six-year-old awkwardness—to arrange them in some semblance of order. "We'll fool everyone and save you from Uncle George."

"But then *you'll* get in trouble."

"Not like you would. Papa might be annoyed, but Uncle George would be . . ."

"I know." Breanna's gaze darted toward Wells, who was now almost upon them. "Are you sure?"

"I'm sure." Anastasia grinned, becoming more and more intrigued by the notion. "It'll be fun. Let's try it, just this once."

An impish smile curved Breanna's lips. "A whole hour or two to speak out like you do. I can hardly wait."

"Don't wait," Anastasia hissed. "Start now." So saying, she lowered her chin a notch, clasping the folds of her gown between nervous fingers in a gesture that was typically Breanna. "Hello, Wells," she greeted the butler.

"Where have you two been? I've looked everywhere for you." Wells's eyes, behind heavy spectacles, flickered from Anastasia to Breanna—who had thrown back her shoulders and assumed Anastasia's more brazen stance. "All of us, most particularly your grandfather, have been worried sick. . . . Oh, no." Seeing the condition of Breanna's gown, Wells's long, angular features tensed.

"It's not as bad as it looks, Wells," Breanna assured him with one of Anastasia's confident smiles. "It was only a little trip and a littler fall."

A rueful nod. "You're right, Miss Stacie," he agreed. "It could have been worse. It could be Miss Breanna who'd taken the spill. I shudder to think what the outcome of *that* would have been. Now then . . ." He waved them toward the dining room, frowning as he became aware of the heavy silence emanating from within. "Hurry. Tell them you're all right. It will certainly brighten your grandfather's birthday."

With an uneasy glance in that direction, he scooted off, retracing his steps to the entranceway.

The girls' eyes met, and they grinned.

"We fooled him," Breanna murmured in wonder. *"No one* fools Wells."

"No one but us," Anastasia said with great satisfaction. She nudged her cousin forward. "Let's go." An impish twinkle. "After you, Stacie."

Breanna giggled. Then, head held high, she preceded Anastasia into the dining room—despite the soiled gown—just as her cousin would have.

Once inside, they waited, assessing the scene before them.

The elegant mahogany table was formally set, its crystal and silver gleaming beneath the glow of the room's ornate chandelier. At the head of the table sat their beloved grandfather, his elderly face strained as he looked from one son to the other. At the sideboard, George bristled, splashing some brandy into a glass and glaring across the room at his brother, who was shaking his head resignedly. Henry nodded as he listened to the soothing words his wife, Anne, was murmuring in his ear.

Grandfather was the first to become aware of his granddaughters' presence, and he beckoned them forward, his pursed lips curving into a smile of welcome. "At last. My two beautiful . . ." His words drifted off as he noted Breanna's stained and wrinkled gown. "What on earth happened?"

"We took a walk, Grandfather," Breanna replied, playing the part of Anastasia to perfection. "We were bored. So we went exploring. We climbed trees. We tried to catch fireflies. It was my idea—and my own fault that I fell. I forgot all about the time, and I was rushing too fast on my way back. I didn't see the mud puddle."

The Viscount Medford's lips twitched. "I see," he replied evenly.

Anastasia walked sedately to her grandfather's side. "We apologize, Grandfather," she said, intentionally using Breanna's sweet tone and respectful gaze. "Stacie and I were having fun. But it is your birthday. And we should never have left the manor."

"Nonsense, my dear." He leaned over and caressed his granddaughter's cheek. His insightful green gaze swept over her, his eyes surrounded by the tiny lines that heralded sixty years of life. Then he shifted to assess her cousin's more rumpled state. "You're welcome to explore to your hearts' content. The only reason for our concern was that it's becoming quite dark and neither of you knows your way around Medford's vast grounds. But now that you're here, no apology is necessary." He cleared his throat. "Anastasia, are you hurt?" he asked Breanna.

"No, Grandfather." Breanna shot him one of Anastasia's bold, infectious grins. *"I'm* not hurt. But my gown is."

"So I noticed." The viscount looked more and more as if he were biting back laughter. "How did you fall?"

"I slipped and landed in a puddle. As I said, I was in too much of a hurry."

"Aren't you always?" George muttered, abandoning the sideboard and marching over to the table. Purposefully, he ignored the girl he assumed to be his niece, instead gesturing for his daughter—or at the least the girl he thought to be his daughter—to take the chair beside him. "Sit, Breanna. You've already delayed our meal long enough." A biting pause. "Perhaps your cousin should change her clothes before she dines?" he inquired, inclining his head to give his brother a pointed look.

"Papa? Mama?" Breanna glanced at her uncle Henry and aunt Anne. "Would you prefer I change?"

Anastasia's father shook his head. "I don't think that will be necessary."

"Darling," Anne inserted, her brows drawn in concern, "are you sure you aren't hurt?"

"Positive," Breanna assured her with that offhanded shrug Anastasia always gave. "Just clumsy. I really am sorry."

"Never mind," the viscount interrupted, gesturing for the girls to be seated. "Dirty or not, you're a welcome addition to the table." He tossed a disapproving scowl in George's direction. "A breath of fresh air, given the disagreeable nature of the conversation."

"It wasn't a conversation," George replied tersely. "It was an argument."

"When isn't it?" his father countered, shoving a shock of hair—once auburn, now white—off his forehead. "Let's change the subject while we enjoy the fine meal Mrs. Rhodes has prepared."

Despite his urging, the meal, however delicious, passed in stony silence, the only sound that of the clinking glassware and china.

After an hour, which seemed more like an eternity, the viscount placed his napkin on the table and folded his hands before him. "I invited you all here tonight to celebrate. Not only my birthday, but what it represents: our family and its legacy."

"Colby and Sons," George clarified, his green eyes lighting up.

"I wasn't referring to the business," his father replied, sadness making his shoulders droop, his already lined face growing even older, more weary. "At least not in the economic sense. I was referring to us and the unity of our family—not only now, but in years to come."

"All of which is integrally tied to our company and its profits." George sat up straight, his jaw clenched in annoyance. "The problem is, I'm the only one honest enough to admit that's what business—*and* this family—are all about: money and status."

Viscount Medford sighed. "I'm not denying the pride I feel for Colby and Sons. We've all worked hard to make it thrive. But that doesn't mean I've forgotten what's important. I only wish you hadn't either. I'd hoped . . ." His glance flickered across the table, first to Anastasia, then to Breanna. "Never mind." Abruptly, he pushed back his chair. "Let's take our brandy in the library."

Anne rose gracefully. "I'll get the girls ready for bed."

"We won't be staying," George said, cutting her off, his jaw clenching even tighter as he faced his brother's wife. "So you needn't bother."

She winced at the harshness of his tone and the bitterness that glittered in his eyes. But she answered him quietly, and without averting her gaze. "It's late, George. Surely your trip can wait until morning."

"It could. I choose for it not to."

Anastasia and Breanna exchanged glances. They both hated this part most of all—the icy antagonism Breanna's father displayed when forced to address his brother's wife.

The antagonism *and* its guaranteed outcome.

They'd be split up again soon. And Lord knew when they'd see each other next.

Quickly, Breanna rose. "Breanna and I will wait in the blue salon, Uncle George," she said, still playing the part of her cousin. "We'll stay there until you're ready to leave."

George was too caught up in his thoughts to spare her more than a cursory nod.

It was all the girls needed.

Without giving him an instant to change his mind, they scampered out of the room. Pausing only to heave sighs of relief, they bolted down the hall and dashed into the blue salon.

"We were wonderful!" Anastasia squealed, plopping onto the sofa. "Even *I* wasn't sure who was who after a while."

Breanna laughed softly. "Nor I," she agreed, squirming onto the cushion alongside her cousin.

"Let's make a pact," Anastasia piped up suddenly. "Whenever we're together and one of us gets in trouble—the kind of trouble that would go away if people believed I was you or you were me—let's switch places like we did tonight. Okay?"

After a brief instant of consideration, Breanna arched a brow. "Good for me, but what about you? When could you ever be in enough trouble to need to be me?"

"You never know."

"I suppose not." Breanna sounded decidedly unconvinced.

"So? Is it a pact?" Anastasia pressed, bouncing up and down on the sofa.

Apparently her enthusiasm was contagious, because abruptly Breanna grinned. "It's a pact."

With proper formality they shook hands.

A knock interrupted their private moment together.

"Girls?" Their grandfather entered the salon, closing the door behind him. "May I speak with you both for a moment?"